Aromatherapy
& Subtle Energy Techniques

Aromatherapy & Subtle Energy Techniques
Compassionate Healing with Essential Oils

Joni Keim & Ruah Bull

Aromatherapy & Subtle Energy Techniques
Compassionate Healing with Essential Oils
Revised & Updated

Book cover designed by Joni Keim
Book cover created by Don Van Amerongen, artist extraordinaire

Photos by Mark Treadwell

Dedications

Joni Keim:
To the remarkable women in my life who have meant so much to me:
My dear mother, Anne Thomas Keim, for her quirky sense of humor, her complete devotion to family and friends, her quintessential mothering, and her superb ability to make a home.
My dear sister, Gini, for treasuring our relationship.
My dear friend, Maryann, for her unfailing strength and support.
My soul mate, Patty, who died much too young and told me to go on.

Ruah Bull:
To my husband, Les, dearest friend and companion.
To all my clients, who have taught me what I know about presence, listening, and compassion.

ISBN: 9781505263879

Contents

Acknowledgments   xiv

Foreword   xv
Dr. Malte Hozzel

Introduction   xvii

Chapter 1: Introduction to Aromatherapy   1
The History of Aromatherapy   2
The Nature of Essential Oils   3
How Essential Oils Affect Us   5
Methods of Using Essential Oils   6
     Inhalation   7
     Bath   7
     Massage   7
     Compress   8
     Body Mister   8
Essential Oil Safety   8

Chapter 2: Introduction to Subtle Energy Therapy   11
Examples of Subtle Energy Therapies   11
     Therapeutic Touch   11
     Polarity Therapy   11
     Subtle Energy Medicine   12
     Earth Energy Healing   12
     Hands-on Healing   12
Our Energy Anatomy   13
     The Primary Energy Centers   14
     The Subtle Bodies   18
The Healing Nature of Compassionate Touch   20
Preparing Your Hands and Yourself   21
     Center in Your Breath   22
     Preparing Your Hands   22
Exercises with Subtle Energy   24
     Feeling Subtle Energy with Your Hands   24
     Sensing the Subtle Bodies   24
     Energy Center Meditation   25

Using Intention and Visualization for Subtle Energy Therapy   27
Using Color for Subtle Energy Therapy   28
The Role of Intuition   29
Subtle Energy Terminology   30

Chapter 3: The Subtle Properties of Essential Oils   33
What is Vibrational Medicine?   33
How the Subtle Properties of Essential Oils are Determined   33
"Listening to an Essential Oil" Exercise   35
The Subtle Properties of Essential Oils: A-Z   37
     Angelica   38
     Anise   38
     Basil   39
     Bay Laurel   39
     Benzoin   39
     Bergamot   40
     Black Pepper   40
     Cardamom   41
     Cedarwood   41
     Chamomile German   41
     Chamomile Roman   42
     Cinnamon, Leaf   42
     Citronella   43
     Clary Sage   43
     Clove   44
     Coriander   44
     Cypress   44
     Dill   45
     Elemi   45
     Eucalyptus   46
     Fennel   46
     Fir, Douglas   46
     Frankincense   47
     Geranium   47
     Ginger   48
     Grapefruit   48
     Helichrysum   49
     Jasmine   49
     Juniper   50
     Lavender   50

Lemon   51
Lemongrass   51
Lime   51
Mandarin   52
Marjoram   52
Melissa   53
Myrrh   53
Neroli   54
Nutmeg   54
Oakmoss   54
Orange   55
Palmarosa   55
Patchouli   56
Peppermint   56
Petitgrain   56
Pine   57
Rose   57
Rosemary   58
Rosewood   58
Sandalwood   59
Spruce   59
Tea Tree   60
Thyme   60
Vetiver   60
Ylang Ylang   60
Choosing Your First Essential Oils   61
Top 12 Basic Essential Oils   62
Top 12 Intermediate Essential Oils   62
Top 12 Advanced Essential Oils   63

Chapter 4:
Using Essential Oils for Subtle Energy Therapy   65
Using Essential Oils with Intention   65
Methods of Using Essential Oils for Subtle Energy Therapy   66
Diffusing   66
Anointing   66
Stroking   66
Misting   67

Applications for Using Essential Oils for Subtle Energy Therapy 67
   Setting Sacred Space 67
      Clear and cleanse 68
      Bring in positive energy 68
      Set up boundaries 69
      Ask for spiritual guidance 69
   Affecting Consciousness 71
   Preparing Yourself 71
   Working with the Energy Centers 72
Essential Oils for the Energy Centers 73
   First: Essential Oils, Common Imbalances, Blends 73-76
   Second: Essential Oils, Common Imbalances, Blends 77-80
   Third: Essential Oils, Common Imbalances, Blends 80-84
   Fourth: Essential Oils, Common Imbalances, Blends 84-87
   Fifth: Essential Oils, Common Imbalances, Blends 87-90
   Sixth: Essential Oils, Common Imbalances, Blends 90-94
   Seventh: Essential Oils, Common Imbalances, Blends 94-97
   Hands: Essential Oils, Common Imbalances, Blends 97-100
   Feet: Essential Oils, Common Imbalances, Blends 100-103

Chapter 5: Helping Ourselves 105
Self-care Questionnaire 105
The Four Dimensions of Well-being 107
   Physical Well-being 108
   Mental Well-being 110
   Emotional Well-being 111
   Spiritual Well-being 112
Self-care Exercise: "20 Things I Would Be Doing If…" 113
Stress: A Part of Life 114
Stress Reduction and Stress Management 115
   Stress Reduction Questionnaire 116
   Stress Management Questionnaire 117
   Three Breathing Exercises 117
   Aromatherapy 118
Emotions Associated with the Energy Centers 119
Assessing Your Energy Centers 121
   Energy Center Questionnaire 121
   Using a Pendulum 125
Balancing Your Energy Centers and Subtle Bodies 126
   Four Dimensions 126

Subtle Energy Therapy   127
Taking Time / Making Time   127
Warm Bath or Shower   128
Helpful Daydreams   129
Creating   129
Nourishment Through Your Senses   130
Being Present   132
Affirmations   132
Actions to Strengthen Your Energy Centers   134
Energy Workouts   136
Tending to an Energy Center   136
Tending Touch   136
Helping Hand   137
Simple Hold   138

Chapter 6: Helping Others   143
Ethical Responsibility   143
Active Listening   144
Basic Hand Positions to Use for Subtle Energy Therapy   145
Open Toes and Close Toes   146
Forehead Spread   148
Simple Hold   149
Filling   153
Combing and Smoothing the Energy Field   153
Giving a Subtle Energy Therapy Session   155
Preparing to Give a Subtle Energy Therapy Session   155
A Session for Relaxation and Stress Relief   156
A Session for Energizing   157
A Session for Relieving Aches   157
A Session to Feel Safe and Secure   158
A Session to Enhance Creativity   159
A Session for Confidence and Self-Esteem   160
A Session for a Joyful Heart   160
A Session for Positive Communication   161
A Session for Mental Clarity and Energy   161
A Session for Spiritual Rejuvenation   162
Ending a Subtle Energy Therapy Session   162
After a Subtle Energy Therapy Session   163
Case Studies with Ruah Bull   164
An Exercise with a Hand Position and an Essential Oil   166

Afterword   167

Appendix I: 169
The Subtle Properties of Uncommon Essential Oils

Appendix II: Quick Reference to Basic Hand Positions   179

Appendix III: 181
Suggested Subtle Energy Therapy Sessions
for Common Imbalances

Appendix IV: 185
"Listening to an Essential Oil" Exercise Fill-In Form

Appendix V: 187
Quick Reference to Key Essential Oils Used
in Subtle Energy Therapy

Appendix VI: 191
Quick Reference to Key Essential Oils for
Subtle Energy Therapy and Energy Centers

Recommended Reading by Chapters   195

Bibliography   199

Index   203

Acknowledgments

Joni Keim:

A special thanks to:

My husband, W. Mark, the magic man, dearest sweetheart, and crazy gentleman, for my extraordinary life with you.

Gail Atkins for her invaluable help editing our original manuscript from a newcomer's point of view.

Malte Hozzel for his contributions, vast knowledge, and wisdom.

My many aromatherapy instructors and colleagues with whom I've shared the allure and delight of essential oils.

My teachers in energy healing, including Margo Bearheart and Phyllis Schubert.

Ruah Bull with whom it has been a great joy to revisit and rework, this, our first book.

Ruah Bull:

Special thanks to:

Becky Green, chosen sister and spiritual friend, for so many things, including my first energy healing class.

Joni Keim, for being my ideal writing partner.

The Christ who came to me in a shamanic journey, and who taught me that I can follow Him and use these energy and aromatherapy healing techniques as part of the Christian path.

The Holy Mystery, Creator of all life, this beautiful planet, and the gift of plants.

Foreword

Joni Keim and Ruah Bull evoke two powerful healing methods, aromatherapy and compassionate touch, and combine them with subtle energy techniques to create this book of substantial knowledge. It is ideal for aromatherapy and subtle energy practitioners as well as lay people who want to dig deeper into the finer levels of healing, prevention, and self-care. This is more than timely because the physical properties of essential oils have been studied at length during the past two decades, but there has been a lack of the understanding of their subtler workings, and how they might be applied in the field of energy medicine. Joni and Ruah, who are true experts in this area, have contributed to this understanding.

Essential oils and compassionate touch work together in a profound way. In an aroma-touch experience, the frontal and posterior doors of the central nervous system are opened simultaneously, activating an incredible symphony of neuronal connections in the brain, brain stem, and spinal cord. This gives rise to a powerful release of neurotransmitters that helps to dissolve our life traumas.

The essential oils are concentrated energy carriers and messengers that nourish all life from an unseen, infinite reservoir of light. Human love is the best expression of this light on earth and is communicated through compassionate touch. There is no better way for essential oils to unfold their full therapeutic energies than by means of an aromatic-touch experience received in a caring setting, under the warm, loving strokes of gentle hands and a compassionate heart.

A work of this kind corresponds to the shift in modern awareness from the matter- and symptom-orientated understanding of medicine that uses synthetic drugs, to the psychosomatic understanding that takes into account mind-body unity and favors natural and plant-derived medicine. Energy medicine, vibrational healing, subtle body therapies, and aromatherapy are the next steps, taking us toward a "mind-over-matter" understanding which experiences consciousness as being responsible for our psycho-physiological destiny.

This implies nothing less than the recognition that we are more than mere physical bodies. It also implies that we acknowledge the existence of the indestructible energy fields around our bodies that reflect our thoughts, emotions, and memories. More than that, we are responsible for these fields and their ability to contribute to our happiness or suffering.

We have to protect this energy field and, if it is disturbed, we can balance and enhance it through energy medicine and subtle energy techniques. In doing this, we can prevent the disturbance from somatizing and becoming *dis-ease*. This approach is a quantum leap for the western mind, but it is long overdue and catches up with established truths. Ayurveda in India and Traditional Chinese Medicine in China encompass the totality of the patient in healing approaches and emphasize the priority of the subtle energies of consciousness over material, the latter being nothing but a form of contraction or condensation of the subtler, finer levels of life.

Essential oils and compassionate touch, communicated through subtle energy therapy, link back to the inner light of universal love, bridging the gulf between matter and energy, helping to join the banks of separation for moments of unity and bliss.

Malte Hozzel
Naturalist and Procurer of Essential Oils
Provence, France

Introduction

Those of us concerned about health and well-being can be grateful to be living in this unique time when ancient and traditional forms of healing, from all over the world, are being re-discovered and re-claimed to accompany the incredible technological breakthroughs of modern medicine.

This book has combined, in practice, two such forms of healing: aromatherapy and subtle energy therapy. Though each effectively stands alone, they are extraordinary when used together. Each has a rich history, having been used for thousands of years in a variety of cultures for religious, ceremonial, and medicinal purposes. Aromatherapy, the use of aromatics and essential oils, was employed by the early Egyptians, Greeks, and Romans, and is mentioned several times in the Bible. Its status as an alternative therapy began in the 1930s. Subtle energy therapy, also known as energy healing, was used in the form of hands-on-healing or laying-on-of-hands, practiced by the Essenes centuries ago, and has been used by the Chinese, Native Americans, and Christian Churches in ancient times as well as present day. Subtle energy gained substantial recognition in the 1970s when UCLA research conducted by Dr. Valerie Hunt and Roslyn Bruyere proved and measured, scientifically, the existence of it in the human energy field. Today, these two remarkable remedial techniques offer us a way to help ourselves and help each other.

Throughout the text of this book, we use the term *healing* in its true sense. To "heal" is from the Anglo-Saxon word *haelan*, which means, to "make whole." If health is a state of wholeness, then healing is that which promotes, supports, and sustains it. Life's experiences can leave us fractured. Yet, everyone has the potential to recover and transcend into wholeness. This book teaches how to use aromatherapy and subtle energy techniques together to serve this purpose of restoring balance and well-being and to, essentially, heal.

The information in this book includes introductions to aromatherapy and subtle energy therapy. There is a comprehensive reference section of the subtle properties of many available and popular essential oils (an A-Z). Basic subtle energy techniques, how we can help ourselves, and how we can help others are described in easy-to follow directions. There is also a list of specific subtle energy techniques to help common imbalances such as backache, congestion, poor circulation, anger, fear, and grief.

The methods taught in this book are simple, safe, and effective and can be used by anyone of any age. The techniques have been gathered from many years of study and experience to provide a solid foundation.

We are all a part of this extraordinary adventure of re-discovering our natural capacity to heal and be healed. We encourage you to tend to yourself as well as others. Everyone can send healing energy as well as bring comfort to someone else. A good friend recently commented, "Life is a team sport." What a heart-warming concept. Indeed, life's ups would be less joyous, and downs would be more difficult without the support and companionship of our family and friends. We share our lives with many people, and we can help others during their difficult or challenging times, as they can help us during ours.

Whether you simply want to help yourself, are a lay person who wants to help friends and family, or a professional who wants to integrate this work into your practice, come to this experience with the playful wonderment, openness, and innocence of a child. We hope that the information and experience bring you, as it has brought us, great joy.

Chapter 1: Introduction to Aromatherapy

Aromatherapy is the art and science of using the therapeutic properties of aromatic, concentrated plant extracts known as essential oils to promote health and well-being. Related to herbal therapy, it has been used, historically, by many cultures for religious, ceremonial, and medicinal purposes. Today, essential oils are used to treat physical, psychological, and subtle energy (including spiritual) imbalances, and have become increasingly popular as interest in healthy lifestyles and self-care grows.

On a physical level, essential oils are used both medicinally and cosmetically. They are versatile in their applications and have many properties. In a medicinal context, they are used to relieve pain, reduce inflammation, relax muscles, support the immune system, promote wound healing, stimulate circulation, and fight bacteria, funguses, and viruses. The most popular methods of using essential oils are massage, baths, compresses, and inhalation. In France, often recognized as the center for medicinal applications of essential oils, aromatherapy is taught to medical students and is used by both doctors and nurses. They are also sold in pharmacies. Eucalyptus, Lavender, and Tea Tree essential oils are commonly used in medicinal applications.

Cosmetically, essential oils are used to nurture and rejuvenate the complexion. They are a boon to skin care because their small molecular structure allows them to penetrate the deeper layers of the skin (dermis) where they can be truly effective. All types of skin, from oily to dry, can benefit. Essential oils can help to balance glandular activity, promote cellular regeneration, soothe, and calm irritations, and stimulate circulation. They are commonly used in facial cleansers, toners, moisturizers, masks, and mists. Lavender, Neroli, Rose, Chamomile (both German and Roman), and Geranium are popular cosmetic essential oils, providing skin-restorative properties as well as imparting their beautiful aromas.

In a psychological context, aromatherapy is used to help reduce uncomfortable mental states such as stress, sadness, anxiety, and anger, and to promote pleasurable mental states such as calmness, peacefulness, joy, enthusiasm, and clarity. These can be achieved in two different ways: 1) by choosing an essential oil with the correct properties such as Lavender, Chamomile German or Roman, Neroli, or

1

Clary Sage for relaxing and relieving anxiety and 2) by using memory and association with an aroma to re-create pleasant feelings. In the latter case, a pleasant-smelling essential oil is used in conjunction with a pleasant experience, such as smelling Jasmine or Rose while enjoying a stroll in a garden or having a massage. When repeated a few times, the pleasant experience and the aroma merge together in the limbic area of the brain, which deals with emotions, memories, and instinctual drives. When this occurs, simply smelling the essential oil can re-create the pleasurable feelings associated with the pleasant experience. Some people like to use the same massage oil every time they receive a pleasant massage so when they smell the oil, they experience a sense of relaxation and nurturing. An association can be created to relieve stress, fear, or other uncomfortable feelings. Hypnotherapists and counselors who practice guided imagery may use essential oils in this way.

On a subtle energy level, which is the focus of this book, essential oils are used to affect subtle anatomy: the energy centers and the subtle bodies. (Subtle anatomy is explained in detail in Chapter 2.) Essential oils are well suited to assist meditations, affirmations, visualizations, and other transformative techniques that benefit from the subtle energy qualities of essential oils. Used for this purpose, aromatherapy is also referred to as subtle aromatherapy. In Chapter 3, there is extensive information about the subtle properties of essential oils, how subtle properties are determined, and an A-to-Z list of essential oils and their specific subtle properties.

The History of Aromatherapy

R.M. Gattefossé, a French chemist and perfumer, is considered the father of modern-day aromatherapy. In the early 1920s, Gattefossé badly burned his hand in his laboratory, and quickly immersed it in the only liquid available, which was a vat of Lavender essential oil. To his amazement, the burn lost its redness and the pain diminished rapidly. As days passed, it healed much sooner than he expected. He was so impressed with this reaction that he began investigating the medicinal properties of essential oils and dedicated the rest of his life to this research, coining the term "aromatherapy" in 1928.

There was some initial interest in Gattefossé's work, but when World War II erupted, it declined. Real interest began with Dr. Jean Valnet's book, *Aromatherapie: The Treatment of Illness with the Essence of*

2

Plants, published in 1964. A French medical doctor, Valnet was inspired by Gattefossé's research. He used essential oils with antiseptic properties to treat wounds and infections, to fumigate hospital wards, and to sterilize surgical instruments. Two of Valnet's students, Margarite Maury and Micheline Archier, brought aromatherapy to England, and used it for massage and skin care. Madame Maury later became respected for her research on both the physical and psychological effects of essential oils.

In 1977, Robert Tisserand, an Englishman, discovered Valnet's book on a visit to France. He translated it, and published *The Art of Aromatherapy* in 1979, bringing the book to the English-speaking world. This book is now available in seven languages. Interest in the use of essential oils grew in Europe. Germany became known for its scientific and chemical research, France for its medical applications, England for massage and skin care, and Italy for psychological applications. In the late 1980s, aromatherapy gained a strong foothold in the United States, led by Kurt Schnaubelt, Marcel Lavabre, and Victoria Edwards. In the 1990s, The National Association of Holistic Aromatherapy (NAHA) emerged as a strong fellowship of interested professionals and lay people, advocating aromatherapy as both a self-help practice and an adjunct to professional services. Today, there is ongoing interest, research, commercial growth, and professional growth substantiating aromatherapy's applications and effectiveness. Of particular significance, aspects of aromatherapy are currently used in hospitals and the hospice setting.

The Nature of Essential Oils

Essential oils are an extraordinary gift from the plant kingdom. Highly concentrated, they are approximately one hundred times stronger than the dried herb of the same plant. They exist in a variety of colors and viscosities. For example, Bergamot is green and watery while Benzoin is amber and thick. Essential oils will last for many years when properly stored in dark, glass bottles with tight fitting caps, and away from heat and light. Essential oils do not contain fatty acids, so they are not "oily" and for this reason, they do not become rancid. Many are volatile, evaporating into the air if left in an open container. This volatility is why they have also been called *etheric* oils.

The quality and therapeutic properties of an essential oil depend on the plant from which it is extracted, the soil in which the plant is grown, as well as the climate, location, amount of sun exposure, amount of water received, time of extraction, and type of extraction. Essential oils can be effective when they are pure and unadulterated, and extracted from plants that have been properly grown, harvested, and extracted. Some plants produce an abundance of essential oils while others produce very little. Most essential oils are complex, and their unique, therapeutic properties cannot be synthetically duplicated in a laboratory.

The price of essential oils varies. The concentration of essential oil in the plant, how it is extracted, and supply and demand ultimately dictate its price. For example, Peppermint leaves produce a large amount of essential oil that is relatively inexpensive. Rose pedals produce very little, taking up to three thousand pounds of petals to produce one pound of essential oil, and as a result, it is quite pricey.

Various plant parts produce different essential oils, such as flowers for Rose, leaves for Peppermint, roots for Vetiver, fruit seeds for Coriander, wood for Sandalwood, bark for Cinnamon, and resin for Myrrh. Interestingly, some plants produce different essential oils from different parts of the plant. The bitter orange tree produces three different essential oils: Bitter Orange from the rind of the fruit, Petitgrain from the leaves and twigs, and Neroli from the blossoms.

Essential oils must be carefully extracted at the right stage of plant development with the right method of extraction in order to preserve the oils' valuable therapeutic properties. The method of extraction must suit the plant while protecting the essential oil. The most common method is steam distillation. During this process, the fresh plant is placed in a vessel into which steam is released. The steam and the essential oil rise from the vessel and are condensed. As they flow through a refrigerated coil into another container, they separate into two parts: the oil part known as the essential oil and the watery part commonly known as the hydrosol. Cold expression extraction is used for citrus rinds, which produces an *essence* and not a true essential oil. (However, it is common and acceptable to call it an essential oil.) In this case, the rind is shredded, sometimes mixed with a little water, and then extracted by pressure. Other methods include the use of solvents and carbon dioxide. Experimentation continues looking for new, more effective methods of extraction to obtain an essential oil while preserving its natural and complete properties.

How Essential Oils Affect Us

Essential oils are used to restore health and well-being via application (coming in contact with the skin) and inhalation (odor molecules entering the nose). The most common methods of use are massages, baths, compresses, misters, and diffusers. When applied to the skin, their small molecular structure and attraction-to-oil (lipophilic) characteristics allow some absorption into the skin where they can enter the blood stream through small capillaries, circulate through the body, and be eliminated through the sweat glands and normal body functions. Most essential oils begin circulating about twenty minutes after application and can continue for as long as twenty-four hours. However, when applied to the skin, some of the essential oil evaporates away, so it is not known how much is absorbed.

When the aroma of an essential oil is inhaled through the nose, certain odor molecules enter the lungs and others travel to the brain. If in the lungs, the odor molecules enter the blood stream and circulate through the body, as described above. Those traveling to the brain are perceived by our sense of smell and have a profound effect, producing emotional responses, memories, instinctual drives, and even affecting glandular functions via the hypothalamus. Anthropologist Lauren Van Der Post said, "Scent . . . is not only biologically the oldest but also the most evocative of all our senses. It goes deeper than conscious thought or organized memory and has a will of its own which human imagination is compelled to obey."

When an aroma enters the nose, it goes through three stages, all happening in a split second.

1. Reception: Odor molecules bind to the *olfactory epithelium* inside the top of the nose. The epithelium contains more than ten million nerve endings that respond to specific aromatic molecules.

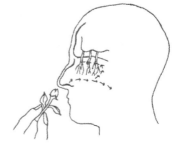

2. Transmission: Nerve impulses are sent to the *olfactory bulb* at the base of the brain, which then sends impulses to the *cerebral cortex* and the *limbic system*. Nerve messages from our sense of smell travel faster to the brain than those from any of our other senses.

3. Perception: The message is received by the limbic system. It consists primarily of the *amygdala*, which deals with instinctual behavior, emotions, memories; the *hypothalamus*, which controls the autonomic nervous system, body temperature, hunger, and thirst; and the *pituitary gland*, which receives messages from the hypothalamus and sends chemical messengers into the blood, releasing hormones that regulate body functions.

Essential oils may be selected for therapeutic purposes based on their chemical make-up. The chemical constituents in an essential oil are responsible for many of its properties and purposes, having unique capabilities and producing effects that can calm, sedate, stimulate, regenerate, reduce inflammation, or inhibit bacteria. For example, oxides have expectorant qualities, making them useful for colds and congestion, and are found in Tea Tree, Rosemary, and Eucalyptus essential oils. Aldehydes reduce inflammation and are calming, and are found in Lemongrass, Lemon Verbena, and Melissa. Esters are a valuable group of components that balance and soothe, and are present in Lavender, Clary Sage, Geranium, and Chamomile Roman. When essential oils are correctly chosen, the desired results based on their properties can be achieved.

The subtle energy nature of essential oils makes them useful for subtle energy therapy. In this case, subtle energy imbalances are addressed. The subtle energy qualities are not based on the chemical constituents of the oil alone. They are based on a variety of information, which will be discussed further in Chapter 3.

Methods of Using Essential Oils

As a rule, when applied to the skin, essential oils are diluted in a carrier oil before use because they are concentrated and can be irritating if used full strength. Carrier oils are plant oils and include jojoba, fractionated coconut, olive, and sweet almond. There are others, but these are ones that are commonly used. The level of dilution depends on the size of the area of skin to which it will be applied, which essential oil is used, the purpose and desired results, and the condition of the skin to which it is applied. Some essential oils and particular situations call for using the essential oils undiluted (neat). A drop of Lavender might be applied to an insect bite or small burn, and a drop of Tea Tree might be applied for fungal infections.

There are many ways to use essential oils. The most common are inhalation, bath, massage, compress, and body mister.

Inhalation

During inhalation, the aromatic molecules of the essential oil travel to the brain and to the lungs, as described above.

Hot water inhalation. Add two drops of essential oil to a bowl of hot water and then cover your head with a towel, close your eyes, and lean over the bowl. Breathe deeply and gently through your nose for about two minutes. For some situations, such as a sore throat, you would breathe in through your mouth.

Diffuser. Diffusers disperse odor molecules into the air by using either cool air or gentle warmth. Follow the manufacturer's instructions.

Direct inhalation. Inhale the aroma through your nose from the bottle or from a tissue on which one or two drops of essential oil has been placed.

Room spray. Fill an eight-ounce mister bottle with water and add ten to thirty drops of essential oil, depending on the essential oil and the purpose. Shake well before each use.

Bath

Baths are especially beneficial because they combine the healing effects of water (hydrotherapy) with essential oils (aromatherapy). They are helpful for muscle discomfort, skin conditions, and emotional imbalance. Mix eight drops of essential oil in one teaspoon of carrier oil and set aside. Fill the bathtub with warm water, immerse yourself, and then add the essential oil mixture. Stir the water around you and soak for ten to fifteen minutes. To relieve muscle tension use Eucalyptus or Marjoram; to soothe your skin use Lavender, Chamomile German or Roman, or Rose; and to relax and relieve stress use Lavender, Frankincense, Clary Sage, or Chamomile German or Roman. If there is not time for a full bath or it is inconvenient, use four drops of the same oils in a half-teaspoon of carrier oil and add to a warm footbath.

Massage

Massage is considered by many to be the best and most effective method of using essential oils for physical and psychological purposes. It is gentle and rhythmic, combining the beneficial effects of touch with the properties of essential oils. Massage relaxes the muscles, and improves muscle tone, circulation, and lymph flow. It also helps release physical tension, which, in turn, relieves mental stress. To make a massage oil, dilute the essential oil in sweet almond oil, fractionated coconut oil, or a blend of vegetable oils. A fragrance-free lotion can also be used. Standard dilution for massage is two percent, using twenty-four drops for every two ounces of carrier oil or lotion. If the skin is sensitive or the essential oil is a particularly strong, reduce this amount to ten drops or less.

Compress

An aromatherapy compress is a damp, folded cloth that has been infused with essential oils and then applied to the skin. (Avoid getting into the eyes.) Either warm or cool water can be used. Warm sedates and relaxes while cool invigorates and stimulates. In a basin of water, put two to five drops of essential oil. Stir briskly and then lay a clean cloth, such as a washcloth, in the water, wring, and apply. Compresses are primarily used for skin care and sore muscles.

Body Mister

Fill a four-ounce mister bottle with water and add ten to twenty drops of essential oil. Shake well before each use and avoid getting into the eyes.

Essential Oil Safety

Because essential oils are concentrated and therapeutically active, they can cause a physiological response, so care must be taken with their use. In many cases, it is the dilution of the essential oil that determines whether it can be safely used. For example, Ginger can irritate the skin if used in a high amount, such as a five-percent dilution. However, in a low amount, such as a one-percent dilution, it can be safely used to relieve muscle fatigue and aches. Some essential oils, mostly from citrus rinds, can cause photosensitivity (a condition in which the skin can burn or become permanently discolored) and should not be used on the skin, undiluted, in direct sunlight.

In addition to the wide range of safe and effective essential oils, such as Lavender, Frankincense, and Tea Tree, there are also a few oils that are not recommended for unsupervised, home use. These include Mugwort, Thuja, Pennyroyal, and Tansy, and there are others. We suggest referring to one of the books listed in Recommended Reading to use as a reference for essential oil safety.

NOTE: In the context of subtle energy therapy, low amounts of essential oils are typically used, usually one percent dilution or less.

The following are standard, recommended safety guidelines for using essential oils:

1. Do not take essential oils internally.

2. Keep essential oils away from children.

3. Keep essential oils away from and out of the eyes. (If this should occur, first put a drop of carrier oil, such as sweet almond, in the eye to collect the essential oil. If no carrier oil is available, rinse extremely well with water.)

4. Dilute essential oils in a carrier before applying to the skin.

5. Avoid applying citrus oils to the skin when the skin will be exposed to direct sunlight. This can cause burning or discoloration of the skin.

6. If you are allergy prone, test the essential oil under a bandage for twelve hours. If there is no reaction, the oil should be safe to use. If there is redness, swelling, irritation, or itching, do not use the oil.

7. If you are pregnant, there are many essential oils you should not use. Use a reference book for this information.

8. If you have a heart condition, there are essential oils you should not use. Use a reference book for this information.

9. If you are taking homeopathic remedies, essential oils may negate their effect. Check with your physician.

10. Do not put essential oils near a flame. They are flammable.

11. If you have epilepsy, do not use essential oils without consulting your physician.

12. If you have asthma, do not use essential oils without consulting your physician.

13. If your skin becomes irritated with an essential oil, apply a carrier oil to the area, wash with soap and water, and then rinse well. Discontinue use of the essential oil.

14. Dilute essential oils in a teaspoon of carrier oil before adding them to your bath. Immerse yourself into the bath BEFORE you add the essential oils.

15. Store essential oils tightly closed in dark, glass bottles, away from heat and light.

16. Care must be taken when using essential oils with children. Use a reference book for this information and avoid essential oils that are high in menthol, such as Peppermint, with children under the age of three.

Chapter 2: Introduction to Subtle Energy Therapy

Subtle energy therapy is a field of therapeutic work that is practiced by laypersons for self-care as well as professionals in a clinical setting. It is a general term for a variety of methods being used today. Though their philosophies, styles, and techniques may vary, they are all based on the same principle, substantiated by quantum physics and neuropsychology, that the world we perceive as solid and material is actually composed of energy, including our bodies.

Subtle energy therapy, then, works with our body's subtle energy—its energy centers and its energy field. Hands and supportive techniques can be used to influence and direct the body's subtle energy in a therapeutic way to promote health, balance, and well-being. Subtle energy therapy can relieve tension and stress, reduce physical and emotional discomfort, boost the immune system, help with preparation for surgery, help with recovery from surgery, and help in spiritual development.

Some subtle energy therapies include Therapeutic Touch, aspects of Polarity Therapy, Subtle Energy Medicine, and the teachings of two highly recognized instructors, Earth Energy Healing with Rosalyn Bruyere and Hands-on Healing with Barbara Brennan. A practitioner in each of these methods offers a brief description below about their area of expertise.

Examples of Subtle Energy Therapies

Therapeutic Touch was developed by Dolores Krieger and Dora Kunz in 1972. "To promote healing, the practitioner centers and aligns him/herself to use universal energy as the means to consciously direct or adjust the receiver's energy. It is done by passing the hands over the receiver's body to ascertain any abnormalities, cleansing the energy field, and then directing and balancing the energy."
—Calvin Davis, certified in Therapeutic Touch, Jin Shin Jyutsu, Reflexology, and Aromatherapy.
For more information: www.councilforhealing.org

Polarity Therapy was developed by Dr. Randolph Stone, DO, DC, ND in the early 1900s. "Dr. Stone studied a variety of therapies, including Ayurveda, yoga, and traditional Western medicine, and integrated them into a new, wholistic health system. Polarity includes body work, nutrition, exercises, and developing a positive attitude."
—Jan Fitzgerald, certified in massage therapy, hypnotherapy, and aromatherapy, and Ph.D. in Educational Linguistics.
For more information: www.polaritytherapy.org

Subtle Energy Medicine is an example of an integrative approach to subtle energy therapy. It is "a method in which the practitioner channels different energy frequencies through their subtle energy body into the receiver's subtle energy system. The receiver takes this energy transmission to revitalize and encourage healing. This system uses an ultrasound frequency that helps the blocked energy of the receiver to open up and receive."
—Margo Bearheart, founder of Transformational Healing Arts Center
For more information: www.issseem.org

Earth Energy Healing, developed by Rosalyn Bruyere, "is a technique that draws vibrational energy up from the earth that is then channeled through the practitioner's body and hands to impact the physical and etheric body of the receiver. It uses sound, as well as light frequencies to bring the system into balance."
—Ruah Bull, Ph.D., certified in hypnotherapy, energy healing, aromatherapy, and spiritual direction.
For more information: www.rosalynbruyere.org

Hands-on Healing, developed by Barbara Brennan, uses "the body's innate wisdom and natural instincts to move towards health. A healer trained in this method works with the different dimensions of being: physical, auric, hara, and core star. By using laying-on-of-hands, the healer releases blocks, balances, and charges the energy field surrounding the body. This enables one to realign with the creative force which is available to each and everyone."
—Betsy Ginkel, certified in the Barbara Brennan School of Healing.
For more information: www.barbarabrennan.com

Our Energy Anatomy

Subtle energy is produced by our body's energy anatomy, also known as *subtle anatomy*. This anatomy consists of *energy centers* and the *energy field*. The seven primary energy centers are located along the spine from the tailbone to the top of the head. These spinning energy centers are often called *chakras*, a Sanskrit word meaning "wheels of light." They receive, assimilate, and transmit various forms of energy, and play a vital role in our state of consciousness and emotions. The energy centers correspond to major aspects of our lives: survival, sex, power, love, communication, conscious thought, intuition, and spirituality. In the *Sevenfold Journey*, Anodea Judith and Selene Vega write, "None of the chakras function by 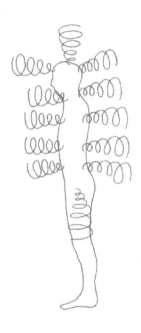 themselves. As wheels spinning at the core of our being, the chakras are intermeshing gears, working together to run the delicate machinery of our lives."

The energy field is made up of levels of energy that permeate throughout the physical body and continue outward from the skin forming an energy structure, which has been referred to as an *aura*. The energy field can extend from a foot to many feet away from the body, the average being about three feet or one's arm's length.

The energy field is generally described as being composed of four to seven *subtle bodies*, depending on the source of information. We use the four-subtle-body model. The subtle bodies closest to the physical body are the densest and have lower vibrations. As the subtle bodies move away from the physical body, they become less dense and have higher vibrations. The subtle bodies shift constantly in response to life experiences and moods—changing in shape, size, and color. They expand with uplifting thoughts and feelings such as joy and happiness, and contract with dispiriting feelings such as fear or hatred.

13

The Primary Energy Centers

Ideally, the seven primary energy centers spin harmoniously together, clockwise. (The orientation for this clockwise motion is from the outside, looking at the body.) Anodea Judith states in *Eastern Body, Western Mind*, "All of the chakras need to be open and functioning in balance with the others to be a fully thriving human being." The shape of their spin should be circular, full, and of equal size and shape to each other. The First energy center's spin, at the base of the spine, points down toward the earth. The Seventh energy center's spin, at the top of the head, opens to the heavens. The others, Second through Sixth, radiate out from both the front and back of the body, in their specific locations. The First, Second, and Third energy centers, located in the lower part of the body, represent the physical realm, and are related to the elements of earth, water, and fire. The Fifth, Sixth, and Seventh, in the upper part of the body, represent the spiritual realm. These triads are joined together and balanced by the Fourth energy center, the Heart, in the middle of the body.

Lesser, or secondary energy centers are located throughout the body. There is an energy center at every joint such as the knees, elbows, and hips. Two important secondary energy centers are the Hands and Feet.

At any given time, an energy center can be blocked or thrown out of balance. Fear is a common reason for this to occur, as well as sudden shock, or repressed emotions or feelings. An imbalance in one energy center can affect the others, especially those closest to it. For example, if you experience sudden grief (Fourth energy center), it can give you an upset stomach (Third energy center) and make it difficult for you to speak (Fifth energy center).

Under stressful circumstances—physical, mental, emotional, or spiritual—the energy centers react and reflect the situations, causing distortions from their balanced states. The spin can speed up, slow down, or change directions (counter-clockwise); the shape can become contorted; and the size can become smaller (constricted energy) or larger (congested energy). All these distortions can cause or represent problems that correlate to the various energy centers. For example, a distortion in the Fifth (Throat) energy center could stem from issues related to communication and may result in physical symptoms such as a sore throat, or psychological symptoms such as difficulty in communicating.

Imbalances or blockages can be eased or corrected by contact with an energy that nurtures, or one that vibrates at the affected center's healthiest vibration. Using subtle energy therapy serves this purpose well and effectively, facilitating positive change.

Following are general explanations of the seven primary energy centers and the Hands and Feet. They include the common name or names of the center, a statement that describes the center's essence, and the location of the center as it relates to the physical body. The concerns of the center (thought of as the duties to which they attend) are listed and the key concept is mentioned first and italicized. If the center is in balance, it reflects the healthy characteristics specified in "Balanced state." Imbalanced states are also noted, providing clues to understanding if a center might be out of balance and requiring attention. Each center provides energy for and is associated with a gland of the endocrine system, as well as other parts of the body. If a center is greatly out of balance, symptoms might be experienced in the associated area. Each energy center responds and relates to a specific color, as listed, benefitting from the color's characteristics. (More information about color follows near the end of this chapter.)

First Energy Center (Root, Base):
Statement: "I am."
Location: Base of spine.
Concerns: *Self preservation.* Connection to Mother Earth, physical existence, survival, health, security, home, food.
Balanced state: Strong relationship with Mother Earth, positive attitude about life, good health, vitality, feeling stable/safe/secure.
Imbalanced state: Disconnected from body, fearful, disorganized, excessive worry, possessive.
Gland association: Adrenals
Parts of body influenced: Urinary system, genitals, intestines, bones, legs, feet, base of spine.
Color: Clear red (revitalizing)

Second Energy Center (Sacral):
Statement: "I desire. I create."
Location: Two inches below navel.
Concerns: *Self gratification.* Sexuality, creativity, desire, reproduction, personal growth, emotions, relationships.
Balanced state: Comfortable with feelings, self-love, enthusiasm about

life, creative, emotionally intelligent and aware, capable of feeling sexual/sensual pleasure.

Imbalanced state: Sexual problems, mood swings, emotionally dependent or detached, feelings of guilt, lack of self-love.

Gland association: Reproductive (ovaries for females, testes for males)

Parts of body influenced: Urinary system, kidneys, reproductive organs, lower back.

Color: Clear orange (energizing)

Third Energy Center (Solar Plexus):

Statement: "I manifest."

Location: Two inches above navel.

Concerns: *Personal identity.* Personality, personal power and will, vitality, self-worth, likes and dislikes, social identity, beliefs, attitudes, activities.

Balanced state: Inner harmony, self-acceptance, confidence, comfortable with life experiences, attract what is wanted in life, attuned to the present, right use of power, warm personality, responsible.

Imbalanced state: Low self-esteem, temper outbursts, stubbornness, hyperactivity, control issues, trying too hard to please, shame, misuse of power, unable to express anger.

Gland association: Pancreas

Parts of body influenced: Digestive system, stomach, pancreas, gall bladder, liver, middle back.

Color: Clear yellow (invigorating)

Fourth Energy Center (Heart):

Statement: "I love."

Location: Center of chest.

Concerns: *Love and acceptance of self and others.* Love, empathy, sympathy, compassion, connects lower and upper energy centers, appreciation of the arts, one's life purpose, love connection with friends and family, good will, devotion.

Balanced state: Warm and sincere, ability to nurture oneself and others, joyful giving, compassionate, altruistic, grateful, peaceful.

Imbalanced state: Love and intimacy issues, anti-social tendencies, grief, depression, difficulty in forgiving, jealousy.

Gland association: Thymus

Parts of body influenced: Circulatory system, heart, lungs, arms, breasts, upper back.

Color: Clear green (regenerating)

Fifth Energy Center (Throat):
Statement: "I speak my truth."
Location: Center of throat.
Concerns: *Self-expression.* Communication (listening & speaking), creativity, time management.
Balanced state: Easily and comfortably able to express feelings, good listener, clear speaker, unselfish, ability to listen to and understand inner wisdom, involved in creative activities.
Imbalanced state: Shyness, fear of speaking, talks too much, selfishness, inability to listen, disconnected from inner wisdom, rushed (feelings of not enough time).
Gland association: Thyroid, parathyroid
Parts of body influenced: Respiratory system, throat, mouth, ears, neck, nose.
Color: Clear sky blue (soothing)

Sixth Energy Center (Brow, Third Eye):
Statement: "I see. I understand."
Location: Center of forehead.
Concerns: *Self reflection.* Intellect, perception, mental clarity, dreams, memory, intuition, understanding, imagination.
Balanced state: Active intelligence, intuitive, good memory, open-minded, open to spirituality, perceptive.
Imbalanced state: Forgetful, impaired vision, overly mental, close-minded, disconnected from intuition, experiences nightmares.
Gland association: Pituitary, hypothalamus
Parts of body influenced: Central nervous system, head, eyes, brain, face.
Color: Clear indigo blue (opening)

Seventh Energy Center (Crown):
Statement: "I am one with the Divine."
Location: Top of head.
Concerns: *Self knowledge.* Sense of oneness, complete understanding, spirituality, faith, higher states of consciousness, divinity.
Balanced state: Balanced with other energy centers, unites inner and outer life, healthy detachment, divinely guided actions, spiritual, thoughtful, wise.
Imbalanced state: Apathetic, fear of death, lack of life purpose, over-attachment, disconnected from spirituality, disassociation with body.

Gland association: Pineal
Parts of body influenced: Central nervous system, brain.
Color: Clear violet (transforming)

Hands Energy Centers:
Statement: "I give, receive, and create."
Location: Palms of the hands.
Concerns: *Service.* Giving and receiving, creating, healing yourself and others, giving and receiving what you want in life.
Balanced state: Gives and receives in healthy ways, trusting, connected to the Heart energy center, creativity flourishes, love flows.
Imbalanced state: Lack of trust, creativity is blocked, over-giving, inability to give or receive, weak or rigid personal boundaries.
Gland association: None
Parts of body influenced: Wrists, elbows.
Color: Warm pink (tending)

Feet Energy Centers:
Statement: "I am grounded. I move with grace."
Location: Arches of the feet.
Concerns: *Being present.* Connecting with Mother Earth, being grounded, receiving and using Mother Earth's energy.
Balanced state: Able to receive wisdom and spiritual guidance, emotionally stable, emotionally responds appropriately and in a timely fashion, present (in the here and now).
Imbalanced state: Emotionally unstable, may lack discernment, emotionally "stuck," confused, inability to concentrate.
Gland association: None
Parts of body influenced: Ankles and knees.
Color: Dark moss green (grounding)

The Subtle Bodies

The four subtle bodies that make up the energy field play a vital role in our health, providing energy for the seven primary energy centers that will, in turn, be used by the physical body. Dr. Richard Gerber, author of *Vibrational Medicine,* states, "It is becoming increasingly clear that it is possible to therapeutically impact upon physical and emotional illness by affecting the higher frequency structures [subtle bodies] which are in dynamic equilibrium with the physical body."

The etheric body lies directly outside of the physical body. It has a direct correlation with the state of the physical body and all its sensations. The etheric body sustains the equilibrium between the physical body and the other subtle bodies and houses an exact energy replica of the physical body, providing a blueprint. This level is strengthened by good health, including physical exercise.

The astral or emotional body lies next to the etheric body. It houses our feelings and emotions, and our relationships with people, animals, plants, our environment, and the universe. It

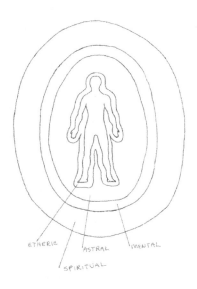

affects the physical body through the nervous, endocrine, muscular, and immune systems. Uplifting emotions (such as love, joy, hope) especially support and expand this level while dispiriting emotions (such as fear, anger, hatred) weaken and contract it. This level is powerful when feelings, both pleasant and unpleasant, are allowed to flow (not repressed). It is strengthened by having good relationships with people, and by giving importance to family, friends, and community.

Next to the astral body, going outward, is the mental body. It houses intellectual function, rational and intuitive thoughts, beliefs, judgments, the conscious and unconscious mind, and memories. This level is positively strengthened by activities such as learning, studying, and meditating.

The outermost level is the spiritual body, which houses our spiritual essence and knowing our life's purpose. It connects us to our spiritual self and emotional experiences of Divine love, spiritual joy, and bliss. The spiritual body organizes the subtle bodies and holds them in association with the physical body. It provides a protective boundary where our energy ends, and the rest of the world begins. This level is strengthened by maintaining harmony in our life, seeking higher truths, feeling connected to a greater purpose, and knowing we are a part of a greater plan.

Rosalyn Bruyere, author of *Wheels of Light*, explains that an abnormality in the subtle bodies can be a warning that something is wrong in the physical body even though there may not yet be physical symptoms. She believes that *dis*-ease manifests first in the subtle bodies on an energy level, and then condenses to manifest in the physical body. If a disturbance is detected and treated in the subtle bodies, *dis*-ease and disharmony in the physical body can be helped or prevented. Existing problems can also be influenced and assisted by working with the subtle bodies. To this end, subtle energy therapy uses the hands with intention to direct subtle and healing energy in and around the body to produce a positive change.

The Healing Nature of Compassionate Touch

"The skin of the human being is an extraordinary liminal boundary where inner and outer realities of body and soul meet. In therapeutic body work there is an exceptional opportunity not only to alleviate physical pain and stress, but also to address the deep feeling and suffering of the soul."
—Patricia Kaminski, *Touching the Soul*

Using hands with the intention to help, promote health, and heal is not new. It is a natural and inherent part of being human and has been used throughout history. What is more instinctual than to put your hand on an aching knee? Or to hold someone who has been hurt? Or for a mother to cradle her crying baby? Archeologists discovered in the Dead Sea Scrolls that the Essenes had trained people in their community to heal with their hands. Native American healers include touch in their ceremonies, and Traditional Chinese Medicine (TCM), in ancient times as well as today, have employed the fundamental principle that hands have the ability to heal.

Using hands in this restorative, benevolent way is a universal language of emotional nourishment that answers a basic, human need. We need to be touched. It is the first of the five senses to develop in human beings, and usually the last to decline. It is an essential part of our well-being and we thrive from the experience of being connected to another. Researchers at the Touch Research Institute at the University of Miami School of Medicine say that a daily dose of touch can be as essential to good health as diet and exercise.

Ashley Montague, author of the 1971 groundbreaking book, *Touching: The Human Significance of Skin*, said, "The communication we transmit through touch constitutes the most powerful means of establishing human relationships, the foundation of experience. Where touching begins, there love and humanity also begin..." Deborah Cowens, author of *A Gift for Healing*, says it is "the most human of all forms of healing, using the hands to reach out in service to another person in a gesture of peace, balance, and love." She reports that, "Studies have shown that those people receiving healing touch have increased alpha brain waves, characteristic of people in a meditative state. Such deep states of relaxation are associated with diminution of stress, improved respiration, better hormonal balance, lower blood cholesterol levels, and heightened immune response."

Many of the subtle energy techniques described in this book are performed with the hands, using them on or around the body to transmit healing energy. They assist subtle energy's unique ability to promote positive change and transformation, and to help manifest intentions. Understanding of the body's energy anatomy complements the hand's ability to give, nurture, and heal.

Beautifully describing hands and their wondrous therapeutic ability, Deborah Cowens says, "The hands are themselves great works of art. They possess beauty, power, and utility. In the hands, raw strength, miraculous precision, and musical dexterity, become one. The hands can build bridges, sculpt stone, type, tie flies, and perform surgery. All the power of our minds, hearts, and souls are concentrated in our hands, which is why they are capable of re-shaping the world. Who can deny that they possess a unique and even awesome power? That power flows from your hands, and you can use it to heal."

Preparing Your Hands and Yourself

Though we all have the innate ability to heal with our hands, it is helpful for you to prepare them, as well as yourself, before working with subtle energy therapy. To use subtle energy therapy with the intention to help yourself or someone else, you must be in a frame of mind that is as positive, relaxed, focused, and supportive. Each of these mental states contributes to the healing nature of subtle energy therapy.

If you cannot achieve this in the moment, it is better to wait until you can. Your hands must also be readied and engaged to send and direct the healing energy, which flows out of the centers of the palms as well as the fingers. The following exercises will help you to feel the energy and help increase its strength.

Center in Your Breath

This exercise helps to relax your body and mind, release unpleasant thoughts, and promote focus. Practice it as often as you can. Once familiar, you will quickly move through the steps, to accomplish the best attitude before working with subtle energy therapy.
1. Sit in a comfortable position.
2. Relax your eyes, letting them rest gently, half closed.
3. Take five deep breaths and notice the way your breath moves in and out of your body. Notice the parts of your body that move with breathing, and the order in which they move. Notice how far the breath moves into your chest and stomach, how much air you draw in, and how much you breathe out.
4. Give yourself the suggestion, "As I breathe out, I release all that is unbalanced and is ready to be released, on a physical, emotional, and spiritual level. As I breathe in, I am drawing in all the energy, and [add what is appropriate for you], that I need.
5. Now bring your awareness into your stomach and let any thoughts you are having float in and out, observing them as if you were watching clouds float by in a big, blue sky.
6. Bring awareness to your breath again and imagine how each cell in your body is being nourished and energized by it. Notice any thoughts and come back to your breath.
7. Let this experience of centering in your breath bring you serenity, clarity, energy, and awareness.

Preparing Your Hands

Practice this three-part exercise as often as you can and use it before you work with subtle energy therapy. It takes only a few moments to complete. If you like, put a drop of Lavender essential oil on the palms of your hands to support the healing energy. Lavender also helps to increase your awareness of healing energy and your ability to feel it. (If you have sensitive skin, dilute the Lavender in a half-teaspoon of fragrance-free lotion or vegetable oil.)

<u>Appreciate your hands</u>:
1. Get into a comfortable sitting or standing position.
2. Take a few deep breaths while you focus, ground, and center yourself.
3. Bring your awareness to your hands. Feel them and appreciate them.
4. Take a moment to reflect upon all the things your hands do everyday. Feel gratitude for them, as they are remarkable!
5. Clear your mind and, again, focus on your hands. Feel and be aware of the differences of each part—the palm, the back, each finger, each knuckle, and each fingernail.
6. Hold your hands together while you visualize them encased in a beautiful pink light, and take three, slow, relaxed breaths.

<u>Activate your hands</u>:
1. Imagine, as you breathe, that you are sending breath directly into your hands. Notice how they may tingle or change temperature.
2. Imagine that, with your breath, you are activating your hands— turning on their energy receptors and preparing them to send healing energy.
3. Take a few moments to feel and experience this sensation.

<u>Gather and prepare energy for your hands</u>:
1. Bring your awareness into your First (Root) energy center. Imagine that it is opening and drawing up the earth's energy as it grounds and replenishes. Let this earth energy move up through your energy centers to the Fourth (Heart).
2. Imagine your Seventh (Crown) energy center opening, and a beautiful wave of pale, violet light pouring into you from above, filling your Heart center, and bringing in spiritual strength, purpose, and guidance.
3. Allow both energies (earth and heaven) to co-mingle with the compassion of your Heart center. In this way, you are tapping into the infinite, bountiful resources of the universe. It is in your best interest to use this energy instead of your own in order to prevent depletion, both from a subtle energy and emotional perspective.
4. Raise all these energies up into your Fifth (Throat) energy center and allow them to pour down your shoulders and arms into your hands. Instruct this energy to keep flowing into and through you until you are finished working with subtle energy therapy.

Exercises with Subtle Energy

Feeling Subtle Energy with Your Hands

Throughout this book, you will read about energy, our nature as energy human beings, and healing with energy. This type of energy has been called "life force" or "chi" in Chinese medicine. This exercise is designed to help you feel and experience this energy as it is sensed between your hands.

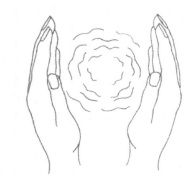

1. Sit or stand comfortably and take a few, slow, deep breaths.
2. Hold your hands about two feet apart, and slowly bring them together. Notice any sensations as they approach, get close, and finally touch each other.
3. Vigorously rub your hands together (this builds energy), and then move them three inches apart, noticing any sensations.
4. Vigorously rub your hands together again. Move them three inches apart, then six inches, then twelve inches, and notice what you feel.
5. From six inches apart, make a small pumping movement with your hands, together and apart, slowly, several times. Imagine an "energy ball" forming between your hands.
6. Experiment with moving your hands closer together and farther apart.

How do you experience feeling the energy? Some people feel a type of tingling or warmth while others sense a thickness, as if holding a balloon or a large cotton ball. However you experience the energy is fine. One way is not more correct or better than another.

Sensing the Subtle Bodies

For this exercise you will need a partner. Because most people cannot see the subtle bodies, this exercise is helpful to practice feeling it. Most beginners are able to sense the etheric body fairly easily with practice. Some people have a "feeling" sensation, others have a sense of "knowing," and still others experience images or colors. Acknowledge your own way of experiencing the energy of the subtle bodies. Again, one way is not more correct or better than another.

1. Have your partner stand or sit comfortably, eight to ten feet away from you.
2. Take a few moments to do the above exercise, "Feeling Energy in Your Hands."
3. Now, hold your hands out in front of you, palms facing forward, in a comfortable position. Slowly approach your partner. As you get closer to their physical body, notice what you feel or sense. You may notice a change in density or temperature or sense a slight resistance. (This usually happens when you reach their etheric body, which is just a few inches away from their physical body.)
4. Continue moving toward your partner. Ask your partner to close their eyes, and to let you know when they can first feel your presence. (This is usually before the actual physical touch.)
5. Begin slowly moving away again. Pay attention to any subtle shifts as you sense the transitions between the four different subtle bodies.
6. Repeat this approach-and-back-away technique a few more times.

Energy Center Meditation

This is an exercise to increase your awareness of your energy centers while you nurture and support each one. Find a quiet, private place. You will need about fifteen minutes, without interruption.
1. Sit in a comfortable, relaxed position with your back supported. Your spine should be as straight as possible.
2. Take a few deep, relaxing breaths and become aware of your entire body. Imagine your whole body comfortable and relaxed.
3. Let your awareness move into your First (Root) energy center at the base of your spine. Visualize, feel, or imagine a clear red light facing down into the earth, spinning clockwise *, round and full. Let this red color become vibrant. Repeat a phrase that nourishes this energy center, and is meaningful to you such as, "I am safe," "I am secure," or "I trust the universe." Feel grounded and connected with Mother Earth and enjoy this sensation.
*Use the following technique to determine which direction is clockwise: Put your right thumb in the center of an energy center of

your choice, such as your Third (Solar Plexus). The direction your fingers are pointing is the clockwise direction of the spin.

4. Move your awareness to your Second (Sacral) energy center, two inches below your navel. Imagine a clear orange light, spinning clockwise, shining out the front and back of your body. Its shape is round and full, and the same size as your First energy center. Repeat a phrase that nourishes this center and is meaningful to you. For example, "I feel my emotions," "I am creative," "I know what I want and desire," or "I deserve pleasure." Feel comfortable with and connected to your creative, emotional, and sensual self.

5. Move your awareness to your Third (Solar Plexus) energy center, two inches above your navel. Imagine a clear yellow light, spinning clockwise, shining out of the front and back of your body, similar in shape and size to the first two centers. Repeat a meaningful phrase such as, "I manifest what I want to accomplish," or "I am a worthy, competent, human being." Affirm your personal power and will.

6. Move your awareness to the Fourth (Heart) energy center in the middle of your chest. Visualize a clear green light shining out the front and back of your body, spinning clockwise. Once again, it is round and full, the same size and shape as the others. Strengthen and affirm this center by repeating a meaningful phrase such as, "I am lovable," "I love others unconditionally," or "I know how to tend to myself and to others." Feel a capacity for compassion and unconditional love.

7. Move your awareness to the center of your throat at the Fifth energy center. Visualize a clear, sky blue light spinning clockwise, radiating out the front and back of your neck. It is the same size and shape as the others. Repeat a meaningful phrase that affirms your capacity to speak, listen, and live with integrity such as, "I speak my truth," "I listen carefully to others," or "I have time to do the things that are important to me." Experience and enjoy being with what is true for you.

8. Move your awareness to the center of your forehead at the Sixth (Brow) energy center. Imagine a deep, clear, indigo blue light shining out the front and back of your head, spinning clockwise, and the same shape and size as the others. Repeat a phrase that is meaningful to you that supports this center such as, "I see and understand," "I have an excellent mind that is both intuitive and rational," or "My imagination supports my creativity and perceptiveness." Appreciate and affirm your mental capacities.

9. Move your awareness to the top of your head at the Seventh (Crown) energy center. Experience a clear violet light, round and full,

spinning clockwise, shining up to the heavens. It is the same size and shape as the others. Repeat a supporting and strengthening phrase such as, "I am one with the Divine," "I am walking my soul path," or "I am open to receiving the wisdom of the universe." Enjoy being aware of your deepest and highest spirituality.

10. Take a few moments to experience all your energy centers, spinning harmoniously together. Sense how your body radiates the clear colors like a rainbow. Visualize the centers becoming the size appropriate for you to return to your daily activities—not too open and not too closed. Look forward to being balanced, knowing your energy centers are drawing in and distributing all the energy they need. Take a few deep, re-orienting breaths, open your eyes, and feel relaxed, refreshed, completely in your body, and fully appreciating who you are.

Using Intention and Visualization for Subtle Energy Therapy

In the context of this book, intention is being clear about the purpose for which you are using subtle energy therapy, every time you use it, while holding the purpose in your mind to direct it. This is based on the premise that energy follows thought and is a form of subtle energy in its own right. Thinking about something is the first step to its manifestation, and there is nothing that has ever been accomplished that was not, at first, a thought.

Your intention in using subtle energy therapy must be positive and restorative. The initial intention sets the stage to start, but it is used throughout to direct its healing energy. An intention statement, or prayer, said aloud or silently, can be incorporated, especially at the beginning, such as, "Let there be healing." A favorite of the authors is, "May [name of person] be healed. May [name of person] receive what they need and may all they receive be for their highest good and the highest good of all."

Visualization can also be used and is another example of how energy follows thought. Shakti Gawain, in her classic book, *Creative Visualization*, says, "Simply having an idea or thought, holding it in your mind, is an energy which will tend to attract and create that form on the material plane." So, when using subtle energy therapy, simply imagine or visualize the desired outcome. For example, if you are working with a stiff knee, imagine it moving and flexing comfortably. If you are working with congestion, imagine the clogged nasal passages draining and becoming clear to allow proper breathing. If working with anxiety, imagine that the body and mind are relaxed and balanced. In this way, visualization is a form of subtle energy and can create reality.

Using Color for Subtle Energy Therapy

Color has been used therapeutically throughout history. When color and light travel through our eyes via the retina to the hypothalamus in our brain, it affects us on physical, psychological, and subtle energy levels.

Colors have a unique vibrational and energy signature that produces a specific effect in subtle energy therapy. It is optional to visualize and send the appropriate color while working with subtle energy therapy as presented in this book, but it is a useful addition and can be helpful in bringing balance and harmony to any area in need.

There is a specific affinity of certain colors with each of the energy centers. Using those correlating colors is the most common usage of color in subtle energy therapy; however, colors can be beneficial for any area of the body to achieve a particular result. The soothing, vibrational qualities of blue can calm an inflamed condition, such as a sprained ankle. Red stimulates and can help in an area that has poor circulation, such as cold feet. Orange can bring cheerfulness to the heart, helping to relieve emotional sadness. Yellow can promote mental clarity, relieving confusion or worry when used around the head. Violet provides a protective boundary in stressful situations when used to fill the energy field.

Following are the basic colors used in subtle energy therapy and their general effects and qualities. Keep in mind that there are infinite hues and shades of colors. Feel free to experiment with color while working with subtle energy therapy for yourself and for others. When possible, ask for feedback from your receiver.

Red: Warming, stimulating, revitalizing. Power, strength, courage. Correlates with the First (Root) energy center.

Orange: Warming, activating, rejuvenating. Enthusiasm, cheerfulness, well-being, optimism. Correlates with the Second (Sacral) energy center.

Yellow: Warming, awakening, inspiring. Knowledge, mental clarity and vitality, joy, happiness, intellectual ability. Correlates with the Third (Solar Plexus) energy center.

Green: Cooling, balancing, soothing, calming, cleansing. Harmony, friendliness, hope, peace, stability. Correlates with the Fourth (Heart) energy center.

Sky blue: Cooling, soothing, calming. Concentration, sincerity, devotion, introspection. Correlates with the Fifth (Throat) energy center.

Indigo blue: Cooling, soothing, calming. Devotion, intuition, integration, present awareness. Correlates with the Sixth (Brow) energy center.

Violet: Cooling, relaxing, inspiring, purifying, restoring. Creativity, humility, protection, spirituality. Correlates with the Seventh (Crown) energy center.

Pink: Cooling, soothing, comforting, nurturing. Tend to others, love, compassion. Correlates with the Hands.

Dark moss green: Cooling, grounding, stabilizing, steadying, comforting. Solid, balanced. Correlates with the Feet.

White: Cooling, transcending, meditative, protective, purifying, transporting. Strength, creativity, stability, virtuous. Related to higher consciousness.

Gold: Warming, strengthening, restoring. Harmony, enthusiasm. Related to higher consciousness.

The Role of Intuition

Using subtle energy therapy helps promote the opening and development of intuition because they are both from the subtle realm. Intuition is the ability to perceive in a way that seems unrelated to the five other senses (seeing, touching, tasting, smelling, and hearing). Psychologist Frances Vaughan, in her book, *The Inward Arc*, says that "intuition [is] a way of knowing that which transcends empirical and rational modes of knowing...given attention, it unfolds spontaneously."

Everyone has the capability to be intuitive. It is a creative capacity of the mind and tends to operate with insightful hunches such as, "I don't know why, but I just had a feeling…" Intuition becomes stronger the more you use and trust it. It is not unusual for people using subtle energy therapy to have strong feelings about changing a technique or even creating a new one. Pay attention to your intuition, and feel free to respond to it. Please note, however, that though intuition is remarkable and useful, like all human faculties, it is not infallible. If you are working with another person, ask for feedback on what you are doing, including that which is based on intuition.

Subtle Energy Terminology

In this book, we use terms associated with subtle energy and subtle anatomy that may be unfamiliar. Following are some of the more common ones and their explanations.

Balancing an energy center is the process of directing an energy center to achieve its optimal functioning—not too closed and not too open. Balancing helps the person remain calm and centered in any situation.

Grounded refers to a healthy, strong First (Root) energy center. For example, when a person is well grounded, they are in the present moment, aware of their body, fully *in* their body, and connected to Mother Earth. They feel safe and secure in the world and their earthly experiences. They love life.

It is best to be properly grounded before using subtle energy therapy. If you are working on someone else, they, too, should be properly grounded. This is important for three reasons.
1) When grounded, the connection with Mother Earth provides the energy that supports and revitalizes the First (Root) energy center, our foundation. By doing this, all the bodies (physical and subtle) are linked, present, and grounded in the physical, and are more able to send and receive subtle energy.
2) People can be disassociated from their bodies and experiences. Rather than being in the present, they are thinking about the past or the future. Being grounded encourages them to relax, be fully in the moment, and be fully aware to experience the deeply restorative, in-the-body experience of subtle energy therapy.

3) If you are working on someone else, grounding helps enable them to provide effective feedback to you. For example, if their back hurts, they may request a pillow for under their knees. Once a person has been grounded, part of their consciousness continues to be aware of the body, even when in deep relaxation.

Linking energy centers refers to the process of connecting certain centers together in a particular way. Both subtle energy techniques and essential oils facilitate this process. Although the energy centers are always energetically linked and working together, there are times when we want to strengthen this connection and the interdependence of two or more centers. For example, if we want to help someone to think more clearly when they feel in danger, our intention is focused on the connection between the First energy center (feeling safe) and the Sixth energy center (thinking clearly).

Connecting with an energy center refers to the process of sending energy and intention into a specific energy center and making contact so the center can become attuned to you. It is similar to tuning forks vibrating together. If the forks are near each other, they will vibrate at the same frequency even if they had previously been vibrating at different frequencies when further apart. In subtle energy therapy, this connection can go both ways—the energy center begins to attune to you, and you begin to attune to the needs of the energy center.

Healthy boundaries mean the energy centers of the body are opening and closing to a degree that is healthy in any given situation. The boundary, which is the outer boundary of the energy field, *allows in* that which nourishes and is beneficial, and *keeps out* that which might be draining or harmful. In daily life, healthy boundaries help people to prioritize, ask for what they need, and protect themselves from being depleted by outside influences.

Chapter 3: The Subtle Properties of Essential Oils

Aromatherapy and the nature of essential oils was introduced in Chapter 1. It explained how essential oils affect us in a wholistic way— physically, psychologically, and subtle energetically. Following is an exploration in more detail about their subtle energy qualities and how their subtle properties are determined.

What is Vibrational Medicine?

Vibrational medicine is a term used to describe the variety of therapeutic practices that influence our subtle anatomy—the energy centers and the subtle bodies. Subtle energy therapy and subtle aromatherapy are both types of vibrational medicine. Interestingly, subtle energy therapy, as used in this book, is linked to the sense of touch and subtle aromatherapy is linked to our sense of smell. The other of our five senses—sight, sound, and taste—also have correlating subtle energy therapies—color therapy, music therapy, and taste therapy. Other examples of vibrational medicine, not related to our primary senses, are homeopathy and flower essence therapy.

Patricia Davis in her book, *Subtle Aromatherapy*, describes the principle behind the effectiveness of vibrational medicine, "Nothing in the universe is still . . . If we look at the body in the most minute detail every one of its millions of cells vibrates with its own life pattern." Describing the exquisite harmony in the movement of cells, she explains, "This harmony is both a reflection of the cell's health and the source of that health, for as long as the cell moves in its ordered dance every function of that cell will take place in an orderly way, and we experience this as a state of health."

If the order breaks down, the function of the cell is disturbed, and physical, mental and/or emotional imbalance can follow. Therefore, the goal of vibrational therapy is to restore erratic cellular vibration to its original, healthy pattern by *persuasive resonance*—that is, by gently coaxing it to mirror the optimal vibrational model.

How the Subtle Properties of Essential Oils are Determined

The subtle (vibrational) properties of essential oils are used in subtle energy therapy for the purpose of influencing cellular vibration, as described above. Their unique subtle properties are determined by evaluating 1) the long-term, traditional uses of both the essential oil and herb of the same plant, 2) the known physical and psychological effects of the oil, 3) the gesture and signature of the plant itself—its appearance and characteristics, and 4) from personal experience.

The aromatic qualities of plants have been used for religious ritual, meditation, and prayer for thousands of years. Aromas were chosen for their ability to promote feelings of oneness with the universe and closeness with God. Dried herbs were burned as incense and the rising smoke was believed to communicate with the deities. As it rose to the heavens, prayers were offered. Frankincense was the most common aromatic used, and is mentioned several times in the Bible, most notably as a gift to baby Jesus. These spiritual connections have been passed down through the ages from ancient Egypt, Arabia, Greece, and Asia, as well as other cultures such as Native Americans.

The known physical and psychological effects of essential oils can be indicators of their subtle properties. For example, on a physical level, Juniper is cleansing and antiseptic. On a subtle level, it is used to cleanse away negativity, clear energy blocks in the subtle bodies, and purify. On a psychological level, Rosemary promotes mental clarity and relieves mental fatigue. On a subtle level, Rosemary has an affinity with the Sixth (Brow) energy center and is used to promote clear thoughts and insight.

Plant gestures and signatures are how the plant expresses itself—a representation of transformed energy from the sun, the earth, and the elements. These gestures and signatures are used to help determine flower essence properties and are useful to determine essential oil subtle properties as well. These gestures and signatures are determined by looking at the plant (or its picture) from which the essential oil comes. What is it trying to say? What is its color or the color of its essential oil? Where does it grow? What is its aroma and size? Does it look hardy or fragile? Is it tall or short? The plant's appearance and character are indications of what it will offer in the subtle realm. For example, Chamomile German essential oil is blue in color. On a subtle level, it relates to the Fifth (Throat) energy center, which vibrates to the color blue. Because blue is cooling, it can be used to "cool" angry words and promote calm, clear communication.

Malte Hozzel, an internationally known naturalist and essential oil specialist, has a unique understanding and appreciation of the plant kingdom. In this passage, he compares the gestures of two plants from which essential oils are extracted, Clary Sage and true Sage. "Look at the huge, green leaves and the thick stem of the Clary Sage with her large mauve and pink blossoms. Clary is incarnated nature, fully there, expansive and strong. Its scent is musky, sweet, and floral. Everything tells us about a balance between material and ethereal forces. It has powerful harmonizing and euphoric qualities, combining in rare beauty both earthly and celestial energies. On the other hand, the true Sage has a thin stem and small, purple-violet blossoms. Its fragrance is warm, fresh, and herbaceous. It has iridescent, fine, grey-blue hairs on the surface of its small and soft leaves. Everything tells us about refinement, subtlety. The life force seems to be drawn towards another dimension. Its subtle, vibrational energies work in true correspondence with the finer energies of our central nervous system."

Lastly, and importantly, is personal experience—including information received intuitively. Because essential oils are used in the subtle realm with intention, their purpose can be designed, directed, and influenced. For example, Rose is an essential oil that promotes love and has a strong affinity with the Fourth (Heart) energy center. However, it can be used with intent on the Sixth (Brow) to assist one in experiencing loving thoughts. It might be used on the First (Root) to encourage love of life. As you work with essential oils in the subtle realm, you may have experiences that indicate a different property than known or described in this book. You may have a strong feeling that an essential oil is not working the way it should, or that it is working differently or better than has been indicated. It is possible for this to happen, so it is important to trust your responses and instincts. In addition, if you are working with someone else, it is important to get their feedback. If you choose to use an unfamiliar essential oil, or want to learn more about a favorite one, try the following exercise.

"Listening to An Essential Oil" Exercise

"Listening to an Essential Oil" is an exercise that can help you discover and understand the subtle properties of a particular essential oil. When working with and exploring subtle properties, it is helpful for you to learn how to use your gut feelings and intuition to gather information. This exercise will help you relax, focus, and "listen" while an essential oil "communicates" with you, especially when experiencing the oil for the first time. This exercise is unique and quite helpful in assisting your intuition to receive information, and the more you practice, the easier, and more natural it will become.

1. Find a quiet place where you will be undisturbed for about twenty minutes.
2. Settle into a comfortable sitting position with your back supported. If, during this process, you need to change position, it is fine to do so. It will not interfere with the exercise.
3. Choose an essential oil you would like to explore and place a bottle of it near you.
4. Take three deep, relaxing breaths, and then follow these steps:
At the count of 1, take a deep breath and lift your eyes to look up.
At the count of 2, exhale and close your eyes.
At the count of 3, repeat a few relaxing words to yourself as you inhale, such as, "Relax, release, let go."
At the count of 4, release your breath with an audible sigh and imagine a beautiful wave of relaxation pouring into you through the top of your head, filling your body with a wonderful sense of calm, as you keep breathing.
5. When your body is full, imagine that the energy centers on the bottoms of your feet open, and any remaining stress or tension flows out of your body as naturally as water running down a drain.
6. Then imagine those feet centers closing to their normal size. Take a moment to enjoy this experience. In this relaxed state, you will be in close contact with your intuitive mind, and you can invite your rational mind to observe the process.
7. When you are ready, pick up the bottle of essential oil and hold it in your hands for a moment to perceive its qualities. Notice any impressions you receive as you hold it. You may sense a color, experience a feeling, or recall a memory. You may detect a texture, or an image may appear to you. Some people hear sounds or music. Some smell an aroma, which may or may not be the aroma of the oil.
8. Write down any of your impressions on a piece of paper. You may not receive any impression at all. Remember, there is no right or wrong way for this process. We all experience impressions in our own way and in our own time.
9. Now open the bottle, put a drop of the essential oil on a tissue, and smell it, letting the aroma fill you from head to toe.
10. With your eyes closed, become aware of the aroma, and notice any impressions you receive. (You may smell the oil more than once, but

not too frequently.) Do you like or dislike the aroma? Are there any places in your body that react or feel affected by the aroma? Is there an energy center that is touched or stimulated? Does it make you feel relaxed or energized? Do you receive any sense impressions such as a color, shape, temperature, or texture? Do you see an image, hear a sound, or recall a memory? Without forcing a judgment, notice any impressions, and jot them down.

11. Now imagine you are engaged in a conversation with this essential oil. Ask the following questions and write down the responses. The responses may come to you from any of your senses—as words, feelings, images, or sounds.

Ask the essential oil:

"What are your subtle properties?"

"With what energy center are you most connected?"

"What are your gifts for subtle energy therapy?"

"What are your spiritual gifts?"

"Is there anything about you that you want me to know?"

Ask any other question(s) that are meaningful for you.

12. When you have finished with the essential oil, feel grateful for its willingness to communicate with you in this way. Take a few deep breaths and count backwards from 4 to a return to ordinary consciousness: 4, take a slow, deep breath; 3, be aware of your body and the room; 2, wiggle your fingers and toes with another deep breath; and 1, feel awake, alert, and refreshed.

Now you have completed the intuitive aspect of "listening" to the essential oil. Be aware that intuitive insights need to be substantiated in both experiment and experience. If you are working with an essential oil, and it doesn't seem to be doing what you expected, go back and "listen" further for more information or clarification. You can communicate and connect with essential oils just as you would with any trusted companion. For your convenience, Appendix IV is a fill-in form that can be photocopied and used for this exercise.

The Subtle Properties of Essential Oils: A-Z

Most essential oils have numerous applications in subtle energy therapy. For example, Sandalwood is grounding when used with the

First (Root) energy center. It increases sensuality when used with the Second (Sacral) and encourages states of higher consciousness when used with the Seventh (Crown).

Following is a list of essential oils, their perceived subtle properties, and their correlating energy centers. Keep in mind that these properties are supported, influenced, and directed by your intention. The key energy center for a particular essential oil is highlighted in **bold**.

Angelica (*Angelica archangelica*)
General: Grounds. Connects us with the angelic realm.
First: Grounds and comforts.
Second: Promotes acceptance of and respect for our emotions.
Third: Promotes personal integrity, strength, and stamina.
Fourth: Promotes compassion and understanding, especially of our own shortcomings. Promotes gratitude.
Fifth: Promotes ability to effectively communicate about spirituality.
Sixth: Promotes inner visions. Helps to balance and protect the mind during meditative, healing states.
Seventh: Connects us with angelic guidance—promotes visits, visions, and messages.
Strengthens spirituality. Helps to align us with our higher selves.
Hands: Promotes the flow of spiritual grace.
Feet: Grounds and stabilizes.

Anise (*Pimpinella anisum*)
General: Clears and cleanses the subtle bodies so that energy can easily move through them.
First: Enlivens the physical body. Promotes a sense of security.
Second: Promotes emotional balance.
Third: Supports the development of personal authenticity. Promotes courage.
Fourth: Supports the healing of a wounded heart.
Fifth: Promotes effective, clear communication—both listening and speaking.
Sixth and Seventh: Clears away old thought forms so that spiritual information can be received. Promotes intuition.
Hands: Promotes the ability to receive.
Feet: Grounds the subtle bodies.

Basil (*Ocimum basilicum*)
General: Brings in positive energy. Strengthens.
First: Promotes a sense of security that eases anxiety.
Second: Promotes emotional strength and responsiveness.
Third: Promotes self-esteem, enthusiasm, assertiveness, and the ability to manifest. Supports personal integrity.
Fourth: Promotes a joyful, heartfelt response to life.
Fifth: Promotes clear, strong, positive communication.
Sixth: Clears the mind. Helps strengthen the ability to concentrate. Improves ability to calmly make decisions.
Seventh: Strengthens the sense of spiritual purpose.
Hands: Supports being of service to others.
Feet: Grounds and stabilizes.

Bay Laurel (*Laurus nobilis*)
General: Clears and cleanses the energy centers. Opens the mind.
First: Promotes a sense of feeling safe and secure.
Second: Helps to balance the emotions. Promotes creativity.
Third: Promotes personal power and confidence.
Fourth: Promotes compassion that comes from deep understanding.
Fifth: Promotes confident and inspired verbal communication.
Sixth: Clears mental blocks and outmoded ways of thinking. Opens the mind to new experiences, thoughts, and perspectives. Supports intuition and inspires.
Seventh: Helps to opens us to spirituality.
Hands: Helps to overcome difficulty in giving.
Feet: Grounds and protects.

Benzoin (*Styrax benzoin*)
General: Grounds. Strengthens, supports, and comforts.
First: Grounds and comforts.
Second: Soothes and comforts difficult emotions. Dispels anger, negativity, and confusion.
Third: Helps to behave skillfully during challenging, emotional times. Promotes determination.
Fourth: Promotes compassion and acceptance during challenging situations. Promotes a sense of peace.
Fifth: Promotes calm communication, especially when angry.

Sixth: Steadies and focuses the mind, especially for meditation or prayer. Helps to bring buried thoughts to consciousness to be comfortably examined and understood.
Seventh: Promotes spiritual strength.
Hands: Supports healing energy.
Feet: Grounds. Encourages walking gently on the earth.

Bergamot (*Citrus bergamia*)
General: Clears and cleanses. Brings in positive, optimistic energy. Uplifts yet calms.
First: Promotes joy of earthly life. Supports love of our physical body.
Second: Promotes positivity and positive relationships. Helps to transform challenging emotions.
Third: Promotes self-love and confidence.
Fourth: Opens the Heart energy center and allows love and joy to radiate. Eases and comforts wounds of the heart, especially grief. Increases compassion for others' suffering. Promotes gratitude.
Fifth: Supports the ability to express compassion and love. Encourages laughter.
Sixth: Calms and clears the mind. Promotes positive thoughts.
Seventh: Helps to strengthen the connection to Divine love and compassion.
Hands: Supports the ability to give positive, healing energy.
Feet: Grounds to promote being comfortable in our life circumstances.

Black Pepper (*Piper nigrum*)
General: Energizes. Clears energy blocks.
First: Grounds and strengthens.
Second: Allows challenging emotions to be felt and let go, especially anger and frustration.
Third: Promotes healthy personal power and self worth. Promotes courage, stamina, and self-control.
Fourth: Clears energy blocks through acceptance and compassion.
Fifth: Promotes assertive and courageous verbal communication.
Sixth: Stimulates the mind. Promotes ability to concentrate. Promotes intuition.
Seventh: Promotes receptivity to spiritual guidance. Strengthens faith. Helps to heal any anger connected with spirituality.
Hands: Promotes the ability to give and receive without judgment.
Feet: Grounds and strengthens the body's energy.

Cardamom (*Ellettaria cardamomum*)
General: Promotes generosity and graciousness with others.
First: Helps us to be open to abundance, while enthusiastically accepting life as it is.
Second: Promotes creativity and sensuality. Warms the emotions. Helps us to see the goodness in people and mankind, in general.
Third: Helps us to be graceful with our personal power. Promotes confidence, enthusiasm, courage, and motivation.
Fourth: Promotes strong yet flexible love. Encourages generosity. Helps to teach others from a heart-centered approach.
Fifth: Promotes caring verbal communication and sharing of wisdom.
Sixth: Clears and opens the conscious mind. Promotes positive perspectives.
Seventh: Promotes spiritual wisdom.
Hands: Helps us to respond to someone in need.
Feet: Grounds and reassures.

Cedarwood (*Cedrus atlantica*)
General: Strengthens and balances. Clears and cleanses.
First: Grounds. Connects us with earth energy.
Second: Promotes emotional stability. Helps to balance our emotions.
Third: Promotes confidence, fortitude, and will power.
Fourth: Strengthens ability to be compassionate and loving.
Fifth: Promotes clear, focused, benevolent verbal communication.
Sixth: Helps to clear and steady the mind. Promotes a strong, calm, meditative, positive state of mind. Supports ability to concentrate, meditate, and receive spiritual guidance. Encourages dreaming.
Seventh: Promotes spiritual clarity and faith. Helps to strengthen the connection with the Divine.
Hands: Supports the ability to receive spiritual love.
Feet: Promotes grounded spirituality.

Chamomile German (*Chamomila matricaria*)
General: Calms and comforts. Gently helps balance emotions.
First: Gently grounds. Helpful during emotional challenges.
Second: Helps to calm and soothe emotions. Helps to calmly feel and understand emotions. Promotes calm understanding of our relationships with others.
Third: Helps to calm and balance our personal will. Promotes patience

41

and calm acceptance of our own limitations. Promotes a positive self-image. Supports the calm pursuit of personal goals.

Fourth: Promotes patience and compassion for our self and others. Promotes acceptance and inner peace. Eases grief and sorrow.

Fifth: Supports calm, gentle, and clear speaking of our emotions and truths. Strengthens.

Sixth: Relaxes the conscious mind. Promotes wise understanding and awareness.

Seventh: Promotes understanding of spirituality, helping to clear spiritual confusion. Helps to feel Divine support during emotional challenges.

Hands: Helps to offer comfort to those in need. Helps to receive and give healing energy.

Feet: Grounds. Helpful during emotional challenges.

Chamomile Roman (*Anthemis nobilis*)
General: Calms and comforts, especially the emotions.
First: Gently grounds. Helpful during emotional challenges.
Second: Helps to calm and soothe emotions. Promotes emotional stability and cooperation. Promotes calm understanding of our relationships with others.
Third: Helps to calm and balance our personal will. Promotes patience and calm acceptance of our own limitations. Promotes a positive self-image. Supports the calm pursuit of personal goals.
Fourth: Promotes patience and compassion for our self and others. Promotes acceptance and inner peace.
Fifth: Supports calm, gentle, and clear speaking of our emotions. Connects with the Seventh energy center to help "hear" and communicate spiritual truths.
Sixth: Calms the conscious mind. Promotes wise understanding and astute awareness.
Seventh: Connects with the Fifth energy center to help us be aware of and communicate our spiritual truth.
Hands: Helps to offer comfort to those in need. Helps to receive and give healing energy.
Feet: Grounds. Supports a healing process.

Cinnamon, Leaf (*Cinnamomum verum*)
General: Strengthens, invigorates, and motivates.
First: Grounds and strengthens.

Second: Supports the understanding of emotions, especially related to past events. Promotes emotional strength.

Third: Helps to strengthen will power, self-control, and confidence. Promotes vitality.

Fourth: Promotes generosity. Encourages compassion towards our past.

Fifth: Supports speaking our truth. Strengthens our ability to verbally communicate.

Sixth: Supports intuition. Helps recover memories.

Seventh: Strengthens our spirituality, especially during times of healing.

Hands: Strengthens our ability to send and receive healing energy.

Feet: Grounds and stabilizes. Helps to restore vitality, especially after a healing process.

Citronella (*Cymbopogon winterianus*)

General: Calms and uplifts. Integrates our spiritual and earthly lives.

First through Fourth: Calms and balances. Connects these energy centers, bringing them into alignment with the upper energy centers and Divine will.

Fifth: Promotes calm, verbal communication. Supports discernment of information received from spiritual guidance.

Sixth: Helps to balance the intuitive right-brain and the rational left-brain.

Seventh: Enhances spirituality.

Hands: Helps us to be open to receive spiritual blessings.

Feet: Grounds and balances.

Clary Sage (*Salvia sclarea*)

General: Calms, uplifts, and restores.

First: Grounds and rejuvenates.

Second: Promotes clarity and understanding of emotions through intuitive insights. Helps to calm and balance the emotions.

Third: Promotes confidence and contentment with achievements.

Fourth: Promotes contentment and joy.

Fifth: Supports calm and clear communication. Promotes laughter.

Sixth: Increases dreaming. Inspires. Supports intuition, strengthening the inner eye to "see" more clearly.

Seventh: Integrates intuition with spirituality.

Hands: Supports giving and receiving abundantly.

Feet: Grounds. Promotes stability as well as flexibility.

Clove (*Eugenia caryophyllata*)
General: Strengthens and promotes action.
First: Grounds, strongly in the present.
Second: Promotes emotional intelligence and appropriate emotional responses. Supports the releasing of outmoded feelings.
Third: Promotes courage, action, self-control, and achievement. Strengthens personal will.
Fourth: Strengthens the ability to act with trust and love.
Fifth: Strengthens clarity of verbal communication.
Sixth: Stimulates and strengthens the conscious mind. Inspires. Assists in recovering memories.
Seventh: Strengthens spirituality. Helps to understand personal experiences from a spiritual perspective.
Hands: Promotes ability to receive.
Feet: Grounds and strengthens.

Coriander (*Coriandrum sativum*)
General: Promotes enthusiasm and optimism. Supports healing.
First: Grounds. Promotes a sense of security.
Second: Promotes creativity, spontaneity, and passion. Promotes emotional warmth, enthusiasm, and optimism in relationships. Helps to heal relationship issues.
Third: Promotes optimism. Encourages confidence and motivation. Helps to manifest.
Fourth: Promotes sincerity and optimism. Helps to heal wounds of the heart.
Fifth: Promotes sincere expressiveness.
Sixth: Promotes imagination and helps to improve memory.
Seventh: Strengthens connection to spirituality.
Hands: Supports healing processes.
Feet: Grounds and assures.

Cypress (*Cupressus sempervirens*)
General: Strengthens and comforts. Helps to cope with change.
First: Grounds. Helpful during times of change.
Second: Helps to comfort and balance the emotions, especially during times of stressful change.
Third: Promotes confidence and patience, especially during times of change. Supports willingness to change. Strengthens will power.

Fourth: Helps to welcome and accept the changes in our lives. Promotes a sense of peace.
Fifth: Supports our ability to listen.
Sixth: Promotes wisdom and understanding.
Seventh: Helps us to stay connected to Divine guidance, especially during times of transition.
Hands: Helps us to remain open to help from others.
Feet: Grounds and stabilizes. Helpful during times of change.

Dill (*Anethum graveolens*)
General: Helps to calm, soothe, and balance emotions.
First: Grounds and stabilizes. Helpful during emotional distress.
Second: Promotes emotional balance and harmony.
Third: Promotes skilled and appropriate assertiveness.
Fourth: Protects against the influence of unpleasant emotions from outside sources.
Fifth: Supports ability to verbally communicate about difficult emotions.
Sixth: Promotes insight and understanding, especially following a difficult situation.
Seventh: Promotes a sense of spiritual nourishment and peace.
Hands: Promotes ability to receive calming energy.
Feet: Grounds and steadies.

Elemi (*Canarium luzonicum*)
General: Grounds. Helps to calm, strengthen, and balance.
First: Grounds. Helpful after deep meditation. Balances the spiritual and worldly life.
Second: Promotes emotional balance and calmness.
Third: Promotes the integration of spiritual values into daily life.
Fourth: Promotes compassion, peace, gratitude, and contentment.
Fifth: Supports clear, calm communication.
Sixth and Seventh: Opens our minds to mystical experiences. Promotes mental peace and clarity. Balances the spiritual and worldly life.
Hands: Promotes positive giving and receiving.
Feet: Promotes grounded spirituality.
Eucalyptus (*Eucalyptus globulous or radiata*)
General: Clears and cleanses. Clears energy blocks and negative energy.
First: Grounds and renews.

Second: Supports appropriate emotional responses, especially in relationships. Helps to balance emotions.

Third: Promotes self-awareness, fortitude, and self-control. Helps to ease the burden of responsibility.

Fourth: Promotes a sense of having "room to breathe" when feeling disheartened or suffocating from too much responsibility.

Fifth: Promotes ability to listen, both internally and externally.

Sixth: Inspires. Clarifies thoughts and opens the mind to new perceptions. Promotes positive thoughts and ability to concentrate.

Seventh: Promotes a clear connection to spirituality and a sense of oneness.

Hands: Promotes healing energy.

Feet: Grounds. Helpful during healing processes.

Fennel (*Foeniculum vulgare*)

General: Helps to protect us from outside, negative influences.

First: Grounds. Promotes a sense of security.

Second: Promotes healthy emotional boundaries.

Third: Protects against negativity. Promotes courage, confidence, self-acceptance, assertiveness, reliability, and motivation.

Fourth: Protects the sensitive and emotional heart.

Fifth: Promotes honest and open verbal communication.

Sixth: Promotes clarity of thought. Helps us to recognize negative influences.

Seventh: Promotes a clear connection to spirituality.

Hands: Protects from taking on (receiving) negative energy.

Feet: Grounds and protects.

Fir, Douglas (*Pseudotsuga menziesii*)

General: Helps to clear energy blocks. Helps to balance emotions.

First: Grounds. Promotes a sense of security and belonging.

Second: Promotes emotional balance and harmony, especially in relationships. Helps dispel loneliness.

Third: Supports a healthy, self-image. Promotes a sense of freedom.

Fourth: Promotes living compassionately. Helps to ease loneliness.

Fifth: Supports effective communication, both speaking and listening.

Sixth: Promotes mental clarity and supports intuition.

Seventh: Promotes a sense of inner unity. Encourages spiritual energy to move through all the energy centers.

Hands: Clears energy blocks to promote healthy giving and receiving.
Feet: Grounds. Promotes stability and flexibility.

Frankincense (*Boswellia carterii*)
General: Grounds. Calms and comforts. Stabilizes emotions. Expands the subtle bodies.
First: Grounds and promotes a sense of security.
Second: Encourages calm, balanced, emotional responses.
Third: Promotes courage and fortitude. Helps to break ties with the past.
Fourth: Promotes sincere compassion and service to others. Promotes acceptance and gratitude.
Fifth: Supports the ability to communicate spiritual truths.
Sixth: Quiets and clarifies the mind. Promotes introspection, inspiration, and wisdom. Promotes a meditative state to better receive and integrate healing energy.
Seventh: Focuses and strengthens spirituality. Helps us to know our spiritual purpose. Connects us with the eternal and the Divine, adapting to our needs. Supports our knowing that we are deeply accepted and loved by the Divine. Helps to heal spiritual wounds.
Hands: Promotes the ability to send compassion through touch.
Feet: Grounds. Connects our spirituality with the earth.

Geranium (*Pelargonium graveolens*)
General: Helps to calm and balance the emotions. Has a nurturing quality.
First: Grounds and supports with a nurturing quality.
Second: Promotes feminine creativity and relaxed spontaneity. Promotes harmony in relationships. Helps to balance mood swings.
Third: Promotes self-esteem, self-love, and self-acceptance.
Fourth: Helps to open our hearts to give and receive nurturing love.
Fifth: Increases capacity for intimate communication and laughter.
Sixth: Supports intuition. Promotes the recollection of old memories. Uplifts the mind.
Seventh: Promotes balanced spirituality, tranquility, and a sense of spiritual protection and nurturing.
Hands: Promotes gentle, nurturing healing energy.
Feet: Grounds and stabilizes.

Ginger (*Zingiber officinalis*)
General: Grounds. Strengthens and rejuvenates.
First: Grounds and supports. Promotes a strong sense of security. Helps to restore energy when physically depleted. Supports prosperity and abundance.
Second: Promotes creativity. Helps to restore energy when emotionally depleted.
Third: Promotes courage, confidence, and optimism. Strengthens personal will and self-control. Promotes a sense of freedom.
Fourth: Helps to motivate courageous service for others. Fifth: Promotes diplomatic, assertive verbal communication.
Sixth: Stimulates the conscious mind and inspires.
Seventh: Strengthens spirituality. Enhances the spiritual dimension of creativity.
Hands: Promotes confidence in giving and receiving.
Feet: Grounds and rejuvenates.

Grapefruit (*Citrus paradisii*)
General: Clears energy blocks. Uplifts and promotes optimism.
First: Helps to be in the present moment. Invigorates and rejuvenates.
Second: Promotes emotional clarity and cheerfulness. Helps to clear "stuck" emotions.
Third: Promotes confidence, optimism, and spontaneity. Encourages self-love and self-acceptance. Motivates.
Fourth: Encourages generosity.
Fifth: Helps us to communicate effectively and positively.
Sixth: Clears the mind. Promotes mental clarity and vitality. Supports intuition. Refreshes the mind and promotes inspiration.
Seventh: Helps us attune to spirituality. Clears energy blocks that interfere with spiritual guidance.
Hands: Helps us to be non-judgmental in our giving.
Feet: Grounds and revitalizes.

Helichrysum (*Helichrysum italicum*)
General: Clears energy blocks, especially those caused by challenging emotions. Helps to let go of emotional wounds and begin healing.
First: Grounds and stabilizes.
Second: Helps to comfortably accept and release challenging emotions.
Third: Promotes inner strength and perseverance. Encourages personal growth.

Fourth: Promotes compassion and patience for self and others. Integrates compassion and spirituality. Promotes emotional healing and acceptance.
Fifth: Helps us to verbal communication to assist a healing process. Promotes creative expression.
Sixth: Helps to activate the right side of the brain. Encourages dreaming. Promotes awareness and understanding. Helps to accept and release painful memories.
Seventh: Promotes a spiritual understanding and acceptance of difficult experiences.
Hands: Promotes healing energy.
Feet: Grounds and stabilizes.

Jasmine (*Jasminum officinale*)
General: Calms, uplifts, and harmonizes. Promote creativity and a sense of wholeness.
First: Grounds and promotes enthusiasm for life.
Second: Promotes joy, love, and harmony. Promotes creative and artistic development. Heightens the senses. Promotes sensitivity and sensuality. Connects sexuality with its spiritual aspects.
Third: Strengthens self-esteem and confidence. Promotes healthy personal power.
Fourth: Warms and opens the heart. Promotes joy and gratitude. Helps us to realize our heart's desires. Calms fear.
Fifth: Promotes creative expression in all art forms.
Sixth: Enhances intuition and creative thinking. Inspires. Promotes insightful understanding. Helps release worry so one can enjoy the present moment.
Seventh: Heightens spiritual awareness. Helps to connect with the angelic realm. Connects spirituality and sexuality.
Hands: Enhances creative and artistic development.
Feet: Grounds and reassures.

Juniper (*Juniperus communis*)
General: Clears unwanted and/or negative energy and uplifts. Clears energy blocks in the subtle bodies. Protects against negative influences.
First: Grounds and protects. Promotes vitality.
Second: Helps to clear accumulated emotional negativity. Helps to protect from negative influences, especially from other people.

Third: Strengthens will power and eases fear of failure. Promotes confidence and self-worth.

Fourth: Helps to protect the heart while still being compassionate. Promotes sincerity and humility.

Fifth: Promotes clear, positive communication.

Sixth: Helps to clear mental stagnation and negativity. Clarifies thoughts. Promotes inner vision and wisdom. Protects our thoughts from negative influences.

Seventh: Helps us connect with and act from our highest ideals. Clears energy blocks on our spiritual path.

Hands: Protects us from absorbing negative energy when touching someone else.

Feet: Grounds and protects.

Lavender (*Lavendula angustifolia*)
General: One of the most important subtle energy essential oils. Balances and integrates all energy centers and subtle bodies. Brings in positive energy. Useful in all energy healing techniques to cleanse, clear, calm, and balance (gently energize or gently relax).

First: Grounds, balances, and supports.

Second: Helps to gently balance and stabilize emotions. Promotes ability to mend relationships. Promotes emotional well-being.

Third: Helps to gently balance personal power.

Fourth: Calms, comforts, and steadies the heart. Promotes compassion, forgiveness, gentleness, gratitude, and acceptance.

Fifth: Promotes wise and benevolent speaking and listening.

Sixth: Helps to balance and integrate the right- and left-brains (intuitive/rational). Uplifts and refreshes. Promotes clarity and awareness.

Seventh: Helps to integrate spirituality in everyday life. Promotes spiritual growth and development.

Hands: Promotes healing energy and sensitivity to healing energy.

Feet: Grounds healing energy to support and strengthen.

Lemon (*Citrus limonum*)
General: Clears and cleanses. Clarifies, uplifts, and invigorates the mind.

First: Energizes and rejuvenates.

Second: Promotes emotional clarity. Helps to clear emotional blocks, such as emotional confusion. Helps to ease fears of emotional involvement.

Third: Energizes and strengthens a healthy, self-esteem. Helps to bring clarity and optimism to personal goals.

Fourth: Promotes joy and optimism.

Fifth: Promotes skillful self-expression. Promotes focus and clarity in verbal communication.

Sixth: Promotes objectivity, concentration, and mental vitality. Clarifies thoughts. Supports and strengthens intuition.

Seventh: Promotes a clear and clean connection to receive Divine guidance. Supports spiritual cleansing.

Hands: Helps to discern what healing energy to send.

Feet: Grounds and stabilizes.

Lemongrass (*Cympobogon citratus*)
General: Clears and cleanses. Calms yet uplifts. Clarifies the mind.

First: Refreshes and renews.

Second: Balances emotions and promotes emotional well-being.

Third: Promotes confidence, healthy personal boundaries, and making healthy choices. Promotes optimism and a sense of adventure.

Fourth: Promotes joy, compassion, and forgiveness.

Fifth: Encourages clear and positive communication. Promotes laughter.

Sixth: Promotes mental clarity and flexibility. Supports intuition. Energizes the mind (though calms the body).

Seventh: Helps us to understand the spiritual meaning and purpose of our choices.

Hands: Supports healing energy.

Feet: Balances and promotes flexibility.

Lime (*Citrus aurantifolia*)
General: Clears and cleanses. Revitalizes and uplifts.

First: Grounds and renews.

Second: Helps to clear unpleasant emotions and attachments.

Third: Promotes confidence and optimism. Helps to clear negative influences from other people.

Fourth: Promotes joy and optimism.

Fifth: Promotes healthy, positive communication.

Sixth: Promotes mental clarity and discernment. Uplifts and refreshes the mind. Helps to release unpleasant memories.
Seventh: Helps to understand a healthy and balanced sense of spiritual "purity." Helps to identify spiritual truths.
Hands: Clears negativity.
Feet: Grounds and revitalizes.

Mandarin (*Citrus reticulata*)
General: Uplifts. Promotes youthful joy and happiness.
First: Refreshes and renews.
Second: Helps to access joyful, innocent emotions, such as of a child.
Third: Promotes enthusiasm and cheerfulness.
Fourth: Uplifts and helps a wounded heart joyfully engage in life. Promotes joy and optimism.
Fifth: Supports communication with our inner child.
Sixth: Calms and refreshes the mind. Inspires. Promotes positive thinking.
Seventh: Promotes spiritual joy.
Hands: Promotes joyful, healing energy.
Feet: Grounds and renews.

Marjoram (*Origanum majorana*)
General: Comforts and calms. Warms.
First: Grounds, comforts, and supports. Promotes a sense of security.
Second: Warms and helps balance the emotions. Promotes the ability to receive helpful emotional support and comfort. Helps to ease fear.
Third: Promotes integrity, perseverance, confidence, and courage.
Fourth: Warms the heart. Promotes sincerity and the ability to give. Helps us to accept deep, emotional loss. Eases loneliness.
Fifth: Promotes sincere communication. Supports healthy expression of grief.
Sixth: Quiets the mind. Unifies the intuitive right and the rational left brains. Helps to recall memories.
Seventh: Helps to deepen faith during difficult times.
Hands: Supports the sending and receiving of comfort.
Feet: Grounds and comforts.

Melissa (*Melissa officinalis*)
General: Calms, comforts, and uplifts. Promotes understanding and acceptance, especially during times of loss.

First: Grounds and balances, especially during difficult times. Revitalizes.

Second: Gently promotes emotional clarity. Helps to support and comfort during times of difficult relationship experiences.

Third: Promotes personal strength. Helpful during times of grief and shock.

Fourth: Promotes love and compassion. Encourages cheerfulness, contentment, and gratitude. Comforts and gently clears emotional blocks from grief and shock. Promotes acceptance, peace, trust, and humility.

Fifth: Helps us to be present when hearing about or expressing grief.

Sixth: Calms the mind. Promotes intuitive wisdom and understanding.

Seventh: Promotes spiritual growth and sense of unity.

Hands: Helps to strengthen healing touch ability.

Feet: Grounds. Help to keep us in the present moment.

Myrrh (*Commiphora myrrha*)

General: Grounds, warms, calms, protects, and strengthens. Helps us let go of the past and move forward.

First: Grounds and restores.

Second: Warms the emotions. Promotes healing of emotional wounds. Helps to bring personal and spiritual desires into alignment.

Third: Promotes fortitude and courage. Helps to empower us to manifest our desires.

Fourth: Promotes forgiveness, gratitude, and a sense of peace. Helps to let go of heartaches. Eases sorrow and grief.

Fifth: Supports confident, wise communication.

Sixth: Promotes meditative states. Supports dreaming.

Seventh: Helps to strengthen spirituality. Promotes spiritual calmness. Assists moving forward on a spiritual journey.

Hands: Connects with the higher energy centers while working with healing energy.

Feet: Grounds the lower energy centers, especially during healing work.

Neroli (*Citrus aurantium*)

General: Brings in positive energy. Calms and uplifts. Links lower and higher energy centers—body and spirit. Clears energy blocks.

First: Renews and promotes love of life.

Second: Promotes a sense of freedom and sensual comfort. Eases fears and anxiety. Links with the Seventh center to spiritualize sexuality.

Third: Promotes confidence, self-acceptance, a sense of personal freedom, and the manifestations of our aspirations.

Fourth: Promotes love, gratitude, and a sense of peace. Helps us to experience joyful love. Eases grief and sorrow.

Fifth: Promotes skillful and compassionate communication. Enhances creative expression, verbally and in the arts.

Sixth: Promotes ability to understand. Unites the conscious and subconscious mind.

Seventh: Promotes direct communication with the spiritual realm. Helps to connect us to angels and feel guided. Links with the Second center to spiritualize sexuality.

Hands: Helps to balance giving and receiving.

Feet: Grounds and balances.

Nutmeg (*Myristica fragrans*)

General: Warms and comforts. Enhances creative responses to life.

First: Grounds. Helpful during creative work.

Second: Promotes creativity. Encourages emotional warmth and comfort in relationships.

Third: Promotes a strong self-esteem. Helps to manifest desires.

Fourth: Promotes a heart-centered connectedness to life.

Fifth: Promotes creative expression, verbally and in the arts. Helps us to communicate our intuitive insights.

Sixth: Promotes and supports intuitive abilities.

Seventh: Helps to strengthen the sense of spiritual presence.

Hands: Enhances creative expression.

Feet: Grounds and comforts.

Oakmoss (*Evernia prunastri*)

General: Grounds. Promotes a sense of security.

First: Grounds. Promotes a sense of prosperity, safety, and security. Helps to integrate earthly and spiritual realms.

Second: Helps to provide emotional protection and support.

Third: Promotes effective and healthy personal boundaries, while promoting confidence and a sense of well-being.

Fourth: Promotes compassion for earth and all of life.

Fifth: Supports skillful communication, especially intuitive information.

Sixth: Promotes intuitive abilities.

Seventh: Helps to integrate the earthly and spiritual realms.

Hands: Supports healing energy.
Feet: Grounds. Helps "spiritual" people to value earthly life.

Orange (*Citrus aurantium*)
General: Brings in joyful, positive energy. Uplifts. Clears and cleanses. Gently clears energy blocks.
First: Grounds and replenishes.
Second: Promotes joy and positivity in relationships.
Third: Promotes self-confidence and an optimistic attitude about personal goals.
Fourth: Promotes joyful love and cheerfulness. Uplifts a heavy heart. Promotes gratitude.
Fifth: Clears energy blocks that interfere with ability to communicate (speaking and listening). Supports joyful, verbal communication.
Sixth: Clears, refreshes, and revitalizes the mind. Helps to connect us to angelic guidance.
Seventh: Represents the joyous light of heaven. Promotes spiritual trust and strengthens a spiritual connection.
Hands: Promotes joyful, healing energy.
Feet: Renews.

Palmarosa (*Cympobogon martinii*)
General: Calms. Supports all levels of healing—physical, emotional, mental, and spiritual.
First: Promotes a sense of security and enthusiasm for life.
Second: Calms the emotions. Supports emotional healing. Promotes loyalty.
Third: Promotes self-acceptance and personal growth.
Fourth: Comforts the heart. Promotes acceptance. Supports self-love.
Fifth: Promotes calm, clear communication. Supports affirmations.
Sixth: Clears and calms the mind. Helps with decision-making. Promotes wisdom.
Seventh: Aligns a personal healing journey with the Divine.
Hands: Supports the receiving of healing energy.
Feet: Grounds and supports.

Patchouli (*Pogostemon patchouli*)
General: Grounds and stabilizes. Calms and promotes a sense of peace. Promotes creativity and sensuality.

First: Grounds, strengthens, and rejuvenates. Promotes a strong connection with the physical body.
Second: Promotes enjoyment of the senses. Awakens creativity. Supports good rapport in relationships. Warms the emotions.
Third: Promotes action. Supports manifestation of personal goals.
Fourth: Helps to open and warm the heart. Strengthens the capacity for heart-felt intimacy and caring for others.
Fifth: Promotes creative and artistic expression.
Sixth: Relaxes a tense, over-active intellect.
Seventh: Promotes spiritual sensuality. Helps to mend spiritual wounds, especially in regard to sensuality.
Hands: Promotes enjoyment of touch.
Feet: Grounds. Helps to connect with the earth's energy.

Peppermint (*Mentha piperita*)
General: Uplifts, awakens, refreshes, and revitalizes, especially mentally.
First: Grounds and rejuvenates.
Second: Promotes clear emotional reactions. Promotes healthy personal boundaries.
Third: Promotes self-esteem, integrity, and ethical actions. Helps to discover personal gifts and strengths. Promotes achievement.
Fourth: Uplifts and renews a heavy heart.
Fifth: Promotes clarity and vitality in verbal communication.
Sixth: Stimulates the conscious mind. Promotes clear perception, awareness, and understanding. Inspires and encourages insights. Helps ability to concentrate. Promotes dreaming.
Seventh: Supports the mental/spiritual journey.
Hands: Supports revitalizing healing touch.
Feet: Rejuvenates.

Petitgrain (*Citrus aurantium*)
General: Brings in positive energy. Promotes optimism. Calms and revitalizes.
First: Grounds and strengthens.
Second: Promotes harmony in relationships.
Third: Promotes self-esteem, self-control, and self-confidence. Encourages trust in self and others. Promotes an optimistic attitude.
Fourth: Uplifts the heart. Promotes trust and faith in the power of love. Promotes the capacity for joy and gratitude.

Fifth: Promotes expressiveness and positive communication.

Sixth: Promotes clear perception. Supports intuition. Helps to recall memories.

Seventh: Provides strength for the spiritual journey.

Hands: Promotes healing energy.

Feet: Grounds. Strengthens trust in the earth.

Pine (*Pinus sylvestris*)

General: Energizes (especially the subtle bodies), rejuvenates, and refreshes. Clears and cleanses.

First: Grounds and invigorates. Promotes a sense of well-being.

Second: Encourages humility and trust in relationships. Helps to break up emotional stagnation. Promotes creativity and emotional well-being.

Third: Promotes self-confidence, self-worth, and self-control. Helps to strengthen unique abilities. Promotes perseverance and strength of will.

Fourth: Helps to replenish the heart. Promotes generosity and trust.

Fifth: Helps to bring clarity to communication, especially when there is confusion.

Sixth: Energizes, refreshes, and clarifies conscious thought. Supports mindfulness. Helps to balance the intuitive right-brain and the rational left-brain.

Seventh: Helps to rejuvenate our spiritual purpose and direction.

Hands: Clears away energy that may have been taken on from others.

Feet: Grounds. Helps to connect us with nature.

Rose (*Rosa damascena*)

General: Brings in positive energy, especially love and compassion. Promotes a sense of well-being. Helps to fill holes in the subtle bodies.

First: Promotes inner vitality and a tender passion for life.

Second: Promotes creativity, passion, and love of beauty. Connects sexuality with the heart. Encourages cooperation and devotion in relationships.

Third: Gently motivates. Promotes confidence and a sense of freedom.

Fourth: Promotes love, compassion, hope, contentment, acceptance, and patience for self and others. Calms and supports. Helps to ease and comfort heartaches. Promotes gratitude.

Fifth: Promotes compassion and wisdom in verbal communication with others.

Sixth: Promotes wisdom, purity of thought, and intuition. Promotes mental freedom.

Seventh: Promotes a close, loving, complete, and devoted spiritual connection. Attracts the angelic realm. Connects with angelic guidance.

Hands: Connects the hands to the heart. Promotes compassionate healing energy.

Feet: Grounds and stabilizes.

Rosemary (*Rosmarinus officinalis*)

General: Clears and cleanses. Strengthens, motivates, and energizes.

First: Grounds and revitalizes, especially during stressful times.

Second: Helps to establish healthy boundaries in relationships. Helps to build emotional strength.

Third: Promotes self-confidence and action. Helps to strengthen will power. Clears away unwanted energy.

Fourth: Promotes strong, pure love. Encourages us to help others.

Fifth: Strengthens affirmations.

Sixth: Energizes and clears the mind. Enhances memory. Promotes clear thoughts, concentration, insights, and understanding. Protects the mind from negative influences.

Seventh: Helps us to remember our spiritual path. Inspires faith. Helps us to receive and understand spiritual guidance.

Hands: Helps us to be able to receive, especially spiritual gifts.

Feet: Grounds and protects. Clears and cleanses.

Rosewood (*Aniba roseodora*)

General: Grounds. Brings in calm, positive energy. Warms the emotions. Helps to clear energy blocks.

First: Gently grounds and calms.

Second: Gently helps us to feel and understand our emotions. Warms the emotions. Promotes creativity and sensuality.

Third: Promotes self-acceptance. Eases the ego's need for control.

Fourth: Warms, calms, and comforts the heart. Promotes gratitude. Helps to ease heartaches and grief, especially from our childhood.

Fifth: Promotes calm communication.

Sixth: Supports intuition and meditation.

Seventh: Gently opens us to spirituality, as we are ready.

Hands: Promotes ability to send healing energy.

Feet: Grounds. Supports a healing process.

Sandalwood (*Santalum album*)
General: Grounds. Calms and comforts. Supports healing on all levels—physical, emotional, mental, and spiritual.
First: Grounds and strengthens sense of being. Promotes a sense of well-being. Links with the Seventh energy center.
Second: Warms the emotions. Promotes sensitivity and sensuality.
Third: Promotes self-esteem and personal strength.
Fourth: Warms the heart and promotes trust and gratitude. Promotes the capacity of the heart to receive healing energy.
Fifth: Promotes calm, wise verbal communication.
Sixth: Quiets the mind. Promotes insights and wisdom. Supports deep meditation and promotes the ability to better receive and integrate healing energy.
Seventh: Encourages states of higher consciousness and spiritual development. Promotes a sense of spiritual abundance. Promotes serenity, peace, and a sense of unity. Links with the First energy center.
Hands: Promotes calming, healing energy.
Feet: Grounds and stabilizes. Promotes grounded spirituality.

Spruce (*Picea mariana*)
General: Clears and cleanses. Rejuvenates. Supports intuition.
First: Grounds and rejuvenates. Grounds intuition so that it is practical and useful.
Second: Revitalizes the emotions. Helps to clear emotional confusion.
Third: Helps to strengthen, empower, and motivate.
Fourth: Promotes compassionate intuition. Refreshes and restores a "tired" heart.
Fifth: Promotes the ability to communicate about intuitive information.
Sixth: Helps to develop intuition and receive intuitive guidance. Promotes objectivity and clarity. Encourages new insights.
Seventh: Helps to open us to our spiritual path.
Hands: Promotes cleansing energy.
Feet: Grounds and rejuvenates.

Tea Tree (*Melaleuca alternifolia*)
General: Strengthens and invigorates.
First: Rejuvenates and energizes.
Second: Promotes emotional strength. Helps us to "let go" of what needs to be leg go of.

Third: Promotes confidence and personal integrity. Strengthens the will and self-control. Promotes ability to change.
Fourth: Helps to protect and strengthen the heart. Helps it to comfortably open in difficult situations.
Fifth: Promotes confident communication. Promotes ability to listen to different perspectives.
Sixth: Supports intuition. Promotes new insights and awareness. Invigorates the mind. Helps to understand different perspectives.
Seventh: Revitalizes and strengthens the spiritual journey.
Hands: Cleanses and renews. Helpful after hands have been used for healing work.
Feet: Grounds and energizes.

Thyme (*Thymus vulgaris linalol*)
General: Clears energy blocks. Strengthens and energizes.
First: Grounds and strengthens. Promotes vitality and well-being.
Second: Promotes emotional strength and warmth. Helps to let go of fear, apathy, and emotions that feel "stuck."
Third: Promotes self-confidence, personal strength, self-control, and courage. Helps to motivate.
Fourth: Promotes a warm and courageous heart.
Fifth: Clarifies and focuses communication. Promotes courage to communicate during difficult times.
Sixth: Promotes mental alertness, focus, and concentration. Counteracts "dreamy" states.
Seventh: Promotes spiritual fortitude.
Hands: Clears and revitalizes. Helpful after hands have been used for healing work.
Feet: Grounds and strengthens.

Vetiver (*Vetiveria zizanoides*)
General: Grounds, strengthens, stabilizes, protects, and calms.
First: Grounds and calms. Promotes a deep sense of belonging.
Second: Promotes emotional fortitude and balance. Protects against over-sensitivity. Calms emotional distress. Helps to keep us steady during difficult times.
Third: Promotes self-esteem and personal integrity.
Fourth: Helps to calm and strengthen the heart. Helps to open, yet protect, the compassionate heart.
Fifth: Promotes wise and loving communication.

Sixth: Calms and steadies the mind. Promotes wisdom.
Seventh: Promotes spiritual calmness and a strong spiritual sense of belonging to the earth.
Hands: Strengthens healing touch.
Feet: Grounds, balances, strengthens, and protects.

Ylang Ylang (*Cananga odorata*)
General: Promotes joy, sensuality, and peacefulness.
First: Grounds. Promotes enthusiasm for life.
Second: Promotes emotional flexibility and calmness. Helps to deepen relationships. Promotes creativity and sensuality. Helps unite our emotional and sexual natures. Dispels anger and fear. Helps to break unwanted emotional patterns.
Third: Promotes self-confidence.
Fourth: Integrates passion and peace. Helps to warm and soften a "hard" heart. Promotes the capacity for joy and gratitude.
Fifth: Promotes calm, warm, and joyful verbal communication.
Sixth: Calms and relaxes the mind. Helps to soften rigid thinking and ideas. Awakens new perspectives.
Seventh: Promotes faith. Helps to open us to the joy of spirituality.
Hands: Helps sensuality to be expressed.
Feet: Grounds and calms.

Choosing Your First Essential Oils

There are many wonderful essential oils to use for subtle energy therapy. The following lists indentify the top twelve basic, intermediate, and advanced oils. Basic oils are indispensable and are usually the first oils to have. They have many general applications. The intermediate oils are a good addition to a basic set. The advanced oils have more specific purposes and are invaluable for certain circumstances.

Your preference for particular oils will develop over time and experience. There is security in using familiar oils, and it is fun to try new ones. Enjoy the exploration.

Top 12 Basic Essential Oils (alphabetical list)
Bergamot: Clears and cleanses. Brings in positive, optimistic energy. Uplifts yet calms. Eases wounds of the heart, especially grief.

Cedarwood: Clears and cleanses. Strengthens and balances. Steadies the mind and promotes the ability to concentrate.

Chamomile Roman: Calms and comforts, especially the emotions. Supports calm, gentle verbal communication.

Eucalyptus: Clears and cleanses. Helps to clear energy blocks and negative energy. Inspires. Promotes mental clarity and positivity.

Frankincense: Grounds. Calms and comforts. Stabilizes emotions. Expands the subtle bodies. Focuses and strengthens spirituality.

Lavender: One of the most important subtle energy essential oils. Balances and integrates all energy centers and subtle bodies. Brings in positive energy. Useful in all energy healing techniques to cleanse, clear, calm, and balance (gently energizes or gently relaxes). Promotes compassion, forgiveness, and acceptance.

Lemon: Clears and cleanses. Clarifies, uplifts, and invigorates. Promotes mental vitality.

Orange: Brings in joyful, positive energy. Uplifts. Gently clears energy blocks. Promotes joy in relationships.

Peppermint: Uplifts, awakens, and revitalizes. Stimulates the conscious mind. Promotes clear perception.

Rose: Brings in positive energy, especially love and compassion. Promotes a sense of well-being. Helps to fill holes in the subtle bodies. Promotes hope, acceptance, and patience. Eases and comforts heartaches.

Rosemary: Clears and cleanses. Strengthens, energizes, and motivates. Clears and energizes the mind.

Sandalwood: Grounds. Calms and comforts. Supports healing on all levels—physical, emotional, mental, spiritual. Supports spiritual development. Promotes a sense of peace.

Top 12 Intermediate Essential Oils (alphabetical list)

Chamomile German: Calms and comforts, especially the emotions. Supports calm, gentle verbal communication.

Clary Sage: Calms, uplifts, restores, and inspires. Supports intuition.

Geranium: Helps to calm and balance the emotions. Has a nurturing quality. Promotes feminine creativity.

Grapefruit: Clears negative energy blocks. Uplifts and promotes optimism. Promotes intuition and mental clarity. Refreshes the mind.

Jasmine: Calms and uplifts. Unites and harmonizes to promote wholeness. Promotes creative and artistic development. Promotes sensitivity and sensuality.

Juniper: Clears negative energy and uplifts. Clears energy blocks in the subtle bodies. Protects against negative influences, especially from other people.

Marjoram: Comforts and calms. Warms. Promotes sincerity and the ability to give. Helps to accept emotional loss.

Neroli: Brings positive energy. Calms and uplifts. Eases grief and sorrow. Links lower and higher energy centers—body and spirit.

Palmarosa: Calms. Supports all levels of healing—physical, emotional, mental, and spiritual. Promotes self-acceptance and personal growth.

Patchouli: Grounds and stabilizes. Strengthens and rejuvenates. Calms and promotes a sense of peace. Promotes creativity.

Rosewood: Grounds. Brings in calm, positive energy. Clears energy blocks. Gently opens us to spirituality.

Vetiver: Grounds, strengthens, stabilizes, calms, and protects. Promotes a deep sense of belonging.

Top 12 Advanced Essential Oils (alphabetical list)

Angelica: Grounds. Connects us with the angelic realm. Strengthens spirituality.

Bay Laurel: Clears and cleanses the energy centers. Opens the mind. Promotes intuition.

Benzoin: Grounds. Strengthens and comforts. Steadies and focuses the mind, especially for meditation or prayer.

Cardamom: Promotes generosity and graciousness with others. Warms the emotions. Promotes creativity and sensuality.

Coriander: Promotes enthusiasm, optimism, and creativity. Promotes emotional warmth.

Elemi: Grounds. Helps to calm, strengthen, and balance. Opens the mind to mystical experiences.

Helichrysum: Clears energy blocks caused by challenging emotions. Helps to let go of emotional wounds and promotes acceptance.

Melissa: Comforts and uplifts. Promotes understanding, acceptance, and a sense of peace.

Myrrh: Grounds, warms, and strengthens. Helps us to let go of the past and move forward. Strengthens spirituality.

Oakmoss: Grounds. Promotes a sense of security.

Spruce: Clears, cleanses, and rejuvenates. Supports intuition and encourages new insights.

Thyme: Clears energy blocks. Strengthens and energizes. Promotes self-confidence, personal strength, and courage. Motivates.

Chapter 4:
Using Essential Oils for Subtle Energy Therapy

Subtle aromatherapy and other techniques used in subtle energy therapy stand alone in their ability to promote and support the well-being of body, mind, and spirit. However, using them together creates a valuable synergistic effect. Essential oils, chosen for their appropriate subtle energy properties, gently yet profoundly amplify the capacity and effects of subtle energy therapy techniques, especially compassionate touch.

Using Essential Oils with Intention

We have discussed *intention* as an important foundation of subtle energy therapy in Chapter 2. Intention remains important when using essential oils for subtle energy therapy. It is necessary to be clear about how you want the essential oils to help you in order to receive their full benefit.

There are two types of intention to consider: focused and general. Focused intention names a specific desired outcome, such as relief from an aching back or earning three hundred dollars more each week. A general intention names an improvement in a more open-ended way, such as feeling more comfortable in your body or experiencing greater financial abundance. You can experiment in each situation to discover which type of intention seems best. In some cases, the specific may feel too limiting, and in other cases the general may seem too vague.

The capacity of purposeful thought (intention) to amplify the healing effects of a substance has been reported by Dr. Larry Dossey in his book, *Healing Words*. He describes experiments in which subtle energy therapists held bottles of water with the intention of sending healing energy into the water. "Samples of the water were added to solutions of yeast cells . . . statistically significant increases in carbon dioxide were observed in the yeast cultures given the treated water."

In another series of experiments illustrating the effect of intention, Oskar Estibany, an energy healer, held in his hands a one percent saline solution, which would usually retard the normal growth of barley seeds. The experiments discovered "...that the damaging effect of the saline could be inhibited if Estibany held the container of saline for fifteen minutes." The conclusion is that positive intention for healing can influence a substance. For our purposes, it intensifies the beneficial, subtle energy effects of essential oils.

Methods of Using Essential Oils for Subtle Energy Therapy

The primary methods of using essential oils in subtle energy therapy are diffusing, anointing, stroking, and misting. There are opportunities to use each of these methods, such as when working with the overall energy anatomy, the individual energy centers, or the subtle bodies. Some of their uses are interchangeable, but each one may be better suited for certain situations. (Some terminology used in this section is explained further in "Setting Sacred Space" below.)

Diffusing: Diffusers disperse the aromatic molecules of essential oils into the air. They are used in subtle energy therapy primarily to clear and cleanse a room or area, to bring in positive energy, to ask for spiritual guidance, and to affect consciousness. There are different types of diffusers available. We recommend cool-air diffusers. Whichever one you use, follow the manufacturer's instructions.

Anointing: Anointing is an ancient practice. It means, "to touch with oil," and has been historically used for protection, devotion, and special recognition. For subtle energy therapy, we may use it in those ways, but we primarily use it for working with specific energy centers or areas of the body. To make an anointing oil, dilute one drop of the essential oil in one teaspoon of olive oil or jojoba. (Or three drops in one tablespoon.) Store in a small glass bottle with a cap. Label it so you know what it contains. The aroma will be quite delicate. Remember, essential oils are used in low amounts for subtle energy therapy. To use, put a drop of the blend on your fingertip and gently touch the area in need with your positive intention. If it is not possible to touch the skin, simply hold your fingertip above the area, in the energy field, from three to six inches from the body.

Stroking: If you are not able to touch the body, stroking can be used. Put a drop of an anointing oil on your left palm, gently rub or pat your hands together. Then rest your hands in the area where it is needed and slowly stroke, without touching the body. Commonly, your hands will be three to six inches away from the body.

Misting: Mists are most often used in subtle energy therapy to clear and cleanse a room or area, and to bring in positive energy. They can also be used to set up boundaries, affect consciousness, work with the energy centers or subtle bodies, or used on your hands before working with the hand positions. Create your mist by putting ten drops of the essential oil in four ounces of purified water in a mister bottle. Shake well each time you use it. Mentally hold your positive intention while misting.

Applications for Using Essential Oils for Subtle Energy Therapy

The four main applications of using essential oils for subtle energy therapy are 1) setting sacred space, 2) affecting consciousness, 3) preparing yourself, and 4) working with the energy centers. Some methods, as described above, are better suited than others for each purpose. As examples, anointing is the preferred method for preparing yourself, misting is a good way to clear and cleanse the area, a diffuser is well-suited for bringing in positive energy, and anointing works well with the energy centers.

1. Setting Sacred Space

We believe that subtle energy therapy, as well as any type of healing technique, is sacred. To acknowledge this spiritual dimension, we suggest you dedicate the room or area in which you are working to that which is greater than yourself—to God, spiritual guidance, spirit, higher power, or however you name that which is sacred or holy for you.

There are four steps to create a sacred space: a) clean and cleanse, b) bring in positive energy, c) set up boundaries, and d) ask for spiritual guidance. You may use a different essential oil or blend of essential oils for each step. However, if you prefer, you can choose a multi-purpose essential oil such as Rosemary or Cedarwood, and as you mist the room, intend that it accomplish all four of the steps.

a. Clear and cleanse. This clears the area of past experiences and their resulting energy imprint and readies it for a new experience. This can be accomplished by misting or diffusing essential oils, with intention. Choose one of the single essential oils or the blend below.

Single essential oils to clear and cleanse: Cedarwood, Eucalyptus, and Juniper are the primary essential oils used for this purpose. Pine, Lavender, Rosemary, and Lemon are also good general cleansers.

Clearing and Cleansing Blend Mist
5 drops Cedarwood
3 drops Lemon
2 drops Eucalyptus
Mix in 4 ounces of purified water in mister bottle. Shake well before each use.
　　　If you want to use this blend in a diffuser, mix the essential oils together and use them according to the manufacturer's instructions. (Do not add them to water.)

b. Bring in positive energy. Just as this suggests, this step brings in positive, uplifting, balancing, peaceful energy to both the area and to the consciousnesses of those present. Mist or diffuse the area with one of the following single essential oils or the blend.

Single essential oils to bring in positive energy:
Bergamot and Orange promote joy, cheerfulness, and optimism.
Cedarwood promotes positivity and strengthens the connection with the Divine.
Lavender balances and promotes positivity.
Neroli promotes positivity and instills comfort and strength.
Petitgrain promotes positivity and optimism.
Rose promotes positivity, especially love and compassion.
Rosemary promotes strong, pure love.
Rosewood promotes positivity and calms.

Positive Energy Blend Mist
4 drops Orange
3 drops Lavender
3 drops Rose

Mix in 4 ounces of purified water in mister bottle. Shake well before each use.

If you want to use this blend in a diffuser, mix the essential oils together and use them according to the manufacturer's instructions. (Do not add them to water.)

c. Set up boundaries. Boundaries are created with the intention of providing protection from negativity or any unwanted influences. Similar to "healthy boundaries" as described in Chapter 2, these boundaries allow *in* that which is beneficial, and *keep out* that which might be harmful. Mist the room or area or apply as an anointing oil to areas in the environment, such as a table, the floor, the wall, or the windows, as you hold the intention of protection. Choose to use one of the following single essential oils or the blend.

Single essential oils to set up boundaries:
Cedarwood strengthens and promotes confidence and fortitude.
Dill protects against the influence of disagreeable emotions from outside sources.
Fennel protects against outside negative influences.
Oakmoss protects and supports emotions.
Rosemary protects, especially during stressful times and in relationships.
Juniper protects against negative influences and clears away negativity.
Vetiver protects, especially against over-sensitivity.

Boundary Blend Mist
5 drops Juniper
4 drops Rosemary
1 drop Vetiver
Mix in 4 ounces of purified water in mister bottle. Shake well before each use.

If you want to use this blend in a diffuser, mix the essential oils together and use them according to the manufacturer's instructions. (Do not add them to water.)

Boundary Blend Anointing Oil
1 drop Juniper
1 drop Rosemary
1 drop Vetiver

1 tablespoon jojoba
Mix well together and store in a small glass bottle with a cap.

d. Ask for spiritual guidance. This is simply asking for help and inspiration from a source from the spirit realm that is meaningful to you. It could be God, guardian angels, the universe, a historic spiritual teacher, or someone important to you who has passed away. Use the essential oils by diffusing or applying as an anointing oil with intention of receiving this guidance. As an anointing oil, place one drop on the Sixth (Brow) energy center and one drop on the Seventh (Crown) energy center. Choose to use one of the following single essential oils or the blend.

Single essential oils for spiritual guidance:
Angelica connects us with angelic guidance.
Bay Laurel supports the ability to "hear" and assess spiritual guidance.
Cedarwood strengthens our connection with the Divine and supports the ability to receive spiritual guidance.
Cypress helps us to stay connected to Divine guidance, especially during times of transition.
Lemon promotes a clear connection to receive Divine guidance.
Orange helps to connect us to angelic guidance.
Rosemary helps us to receive and understand spiritual guidance.
Rose, Angelica, and Jasmine attract the angelic realm.

Spiritual Guidance Blend Mist
4 drops Lemon
3 drops Rosemary
3 drops Bay Laurel
Mix in 4 ounces of purified water in mister bottle. Shake well before each use.

If you want to use this blend in a diffuser, mix the essential oils together and use them according to the manufacturer's instructions. (Do not add them to water.)

Spiritual Guidance Blend Anointing Oil
1 drop Lemon
1 drop Rosemary
1 drop Bay Laurel

1 tablespoon jojoba
Mix well together and store in a small glass bottle with a cap.

2. Affecting Consciousness

Use essential oils to create a positive, healing state of mind while working with subtle energy therapy by diffusing or misting the room. Many essential oils can be used for this purpose. Choose from the following single essential oils, the blend, or from the A-Z list in Chapter 3.

Single essential oils to affect consciousness:
Bergamot to calm and uplift the spirit.
Cedarwood to calm and strengthen.
Eucalyptus to clear and renew the mind.
Frankincense to calm and strengthen our spirituality.
Grapefruit to uplift and rejuvenate.
Lavender to balance and refresh.
Orange to promote joy and optimism.
Pine to energize and refresh.
Rosemary to energize and clear the mind.
Sandalwood to calm and comfort.

Positive Mind Blend Mist
4 drops Bergamot
4 drops Orange
2 drops Eucalyptus
Mix in 4 ounces of purified water in mister bottle. Shake well before each use.

If you want to use this blend in a diffuser, mix the essential oils together and use them according to the manufacturer's instructions. (Do not add them to water.)

3. Preparing Yourself

After the environment has been cleansed and imbued with positive energy, anoint the bottom of your feet with a grounding essential oil such as Sandalwood, Cedarwood, or Vetiver. Then, anoint your hands with Lavender. Gently rub your hands together to help activate their energy and make them more sensitive to working with subtle energy. Anointing your Heart center with Rose brings compassion to the work of your hands.

Grounding Anointing Oil
1 drop Sandalwood
1 drop Vetiver
1 drop Cedarwood
1 tablespoon jojoba
Mix well together and store in a small glass bottle with a cap.

Compassionate Hands Anointing Oil
1 drop Lavender
1 drop Rose
1 drop Bergamot
1 tablespoon jojoba
Mix well together and store in a small glass bottle with a cap.

Heart Center Anointing Oil
1 drop Rose
1 drop Bergamot
1 drop Orange
1 tablespoon jojoba
Mix well together and store in a small glass bottle with a cap.

4. Working with the Energy Centers

Much of subtle energy therapy involves working with the individual energy centers with the intention to bring them into balance. Imbalances in the energy centers may be due to too much energy (congestion), or too little energy (constriction). Essential oils and subtle energy hand positions can help restore harmony and balance to the energy centers by coming into contact with them and vibrating at the center's healthiest frequency. Using the appropriate essential oil makes the hand positions more effective. Many essential oils have an affinity with specific energy centers, supporting and promoting the healthy cellular vibrational pattern of that center.

Essential oils can be used to benefit a specific energy center or energy centers in a group in the following ways. One or more of these methods can be used at a time.

Anointing. Place a drop of an anointing oil on your fingertip, and then touch the energy center in need. If the skin cannot be touched, simply hold your fingertip in the energy field above the center, usually three to six inches from the body.

Stroking. Put a drop of an anointing oil on your left palm, gently pat or rub your hands together. Then rest your hands in the area where it is needed and slowly stroke, without touching the body. Commonly, your hands will be three to six inches away from the body.

Misting. Gently spray the area above the appropriate energy center.

Inhalation. Inhale the aroma of the appropriate essential oil from a drop on a tissue. Hold your hands over the energy center and imagine the aroma filling that center.

Essential Oils for the Energy Centers

Following is a list of the energy centers with information to help you work with each one with essential oils. Included are: 1) essential oils that resonate with each energy center. Those that are starred (*) are especially indicated. This is not an all-inclusive list. It is designed to give you a place to start. See Chapter 3 for more information. 2) Common imbalances of the energy center with suggested essential oils to restore balance. Again, these are suggestions. There are others that you might use. See Chapter 3 for more information. 3) Recipes for essential oil blends that are designed for each energy center. Once you begin working with the essential oils and the centers, you may design your own blends, which we encourage you to do. NOTE: Be sure you like the aroma of the essential oil you choose for yourself. If you are working with others, let them smell the essential oil or blend you have chosen before using it. It will be difficult for them to have a positive experience if the aroma displeases them. If there is a negative reaction, choose another essential oil or blend appropriate for the center.

First (Root, Base) Energy Center
Essential Oils
Cardamom: Grounds and helps us to be open to abundance.
*Cedarwood: Grounds and connects us with earth energy.
Coriander: Grounds and promotes a sense of security and earthly contentment.
Cypress: Grounds and supports during times of change.
Elemi: Grounds and helps balance the spiritual and worldly life.
*Frankincense: Grounds and promotes a sense of security.

Geranium: Grounds and supports with a nurturing quality.
Ginger: Grounds and helps restore energy when physically depleted.
Grapefruit: Grounds to energize and rejuvenate.
Jasmine: Grounds and promotes enthusiasm for life.
Marjoram: Grounds, comforts, and supports. Promotes a sense of security.
*Myrrh: Grounds, strengthens, and revitalizes.
*Oakmoss: Grounds. Increases sense of prosperity and security.
*Patchouli: Grounds and strengthens. Good for people who are over thinkers.
Peppermint: Grounds and rejuvenates.
Pine: Grounds and invigorates. Promotes a sense of well-being.
Rosemary: Grounds and protects, especially during stressful times.
*Rosewood: Grounds and calms.
*Sandalwood: Grounds, comforts, and strengthens sense of being.
*Vetiver: Grounds, calms, and protects. Promotes strength and a deep sense of belonging.

Common Imbalances
Constricted Energy
Disconnected from body: Patchouli, Coriander, Geranium, Frankincense, Rosewood.
Underweight: Frankincense, Marjoram, Jasmine.
Weak physical constitution: Myrrh, Ginger, Grapefruit, Patchouli, Vetiver, Peppermint.
Experiencing life on earth as a burden: Frankincense, Jasmine, Coriander, Patchouli.
Fearful: Marjoram, Sandalwood.
Undisciplined: Frankincense, Rosemary.
Disorganized: Vetiver, Cedarwood, Peppermint, Rosemary.

Congested Energy
Materialistic: Elemi, Marjoram, Vetiver, Coriander.
Overweight: Geranium, Pine, Sandalwood.
Self-indulgent: Geranium, Elemi, Sandalwood.
Ignores needs of others: Coriander, Geranium, Sandalwood.
Sluggish: Myrrh, Grapefruit, Peppermint, Pine.
Quick to anger, aggression: Vetiver, Rosewood, Sandalwood.
Possessive: Frankincense, Pine, Sandalwood.

First Energy Center Blends

A. To integrate body and spirit:
First Center Mist A
6 drops Cedarwood
2 drops Sandalwood
2 drops Frankincense
Mix in 4 ounces of purified water in mister bottle. Shake well before each use.

First Center Anointing Oil A
1 drop Cedarwood
1 drop Sandalwood
1 drop Frankincense
1 tablespoon jojoba
Mix well together and store in a small glass bottle with a cap.

B. To increase basic trust in the goodness of the universe:
First Center Mist B
8 drops Frankincense
2 drops Sandalwood
Mix in 4 ounces of purified water in mister bottle. Shake well before each use.

First Center Anointing Oil B
2 drops Frankincense
1 drop Sandalwood
1 tablespoon jojoba
Mix well together and store in a small glass bottle with a cap.

C. To balance the mind and emotions while grounding the physical body:
First Center Mist C
3 drops Patchouli
7 drops Sandalwood
Mix in 4 ounces of purified water in mister bottle. Shake well before each use.

First Center Anointing Oil C
1 drop Patchouli
2 drops Sandalwood
1 tablespoon jojoba
Mix well together and store in a small glass bottle with a cap.

D. To rejuvenate body and mind:
First Center Mist D
6 drops Grapefruit
3 drops Peppermint
1 drop Pine
Mix in 4 ounces of purified water in mister bottle. Shake well before each use.

First Center Anointing Oil D
1 drop Grapefruit
1 drop Peppermint
1 drop Pine
1 tablespoon jojoba
Mix well together and store in a small glass bottle with a cap.

E. To promote enthusiasm for life:
First Center Mist E
5 drops Jasmine
4 drops Coriander
1 drop Geranium
Mix in 4 ounces of purified water in mister bottle. Shake well before each use.

First Center Anointing Oil E
1 drop Jasmine
1 drop Coriander
1 drop Geranium
1 tablespoon jojoba
Mix well together and store in a small glass bottle with a cap.

Second (Sacral) Energy Center
Essential Oils

Bergamot: Promotes positivity and positive relationships.

*Cardamom: Promotes creativity and sensuality. Helps us to see the goodness in other people.

Chamomile German or Roman: Helps to calm and soothe emotions. Promotes cooperation in relationships.

*Coriander: Promotes creativity, spontaneity, and passion. Promotes warmth and optimism in relationships.

*Dill: Promotes emotional balance and harmony.

*Geranium: Promotes feminine creativity and relaxed spontaneity. Helps to balance moods swings.

Ginger: Promotes creativity. Helps restore energy when emotionally depleted.

*Jasmine: Promotes joy, love, and harmony. Promotes creativity and artistic development. Promotes sensitivity and sensuality. Connects spirituality and sexuality.

*Juniper: Helps to clear away emotional negativity. Helps to protect from unpleasant emotional influences.

Lavender: Promotes a sense of emotional balance and well-being. Promotes ability to mend relationships.

Mandarin: Helps to access joyful, innocent emotions, such as of a child.

*Nutmeg: Promotes creativity. Promotes emotional warmth and comfort in relationships.

*Orange: Promotes joy and positivity in relationships and radiant warmth in sexuality.

Patchouli: Promotes enjoyment of the senses and awakening of creativity.

*Rose: Promotes creativity, passion, and love of beauty. Connects sexuality with the heart.

Rosemary: Helps to build emotional strength and healthy boundaries in relationships.

Sandalwood: Warms the emotions. Promotes sensitivity and sensuality.

Tea Tree: Helps to strengthen the emotions. Helps us to "let go" of what needs to be let go of.

Vetiver: Protects against over-sensitivity. Calms emotional distress.

*Ylang Ylang: Promotes emotional flexibility. Helps dispel anger and fear. Helps to deepen relationships. Promotes sensuality. Helps unite our emotional and sexual natures.

<u>Common Imbalances</u>
Constricted Energy
Suppressed sexual desires: Sandalwood, Rose, Ylang Ylang, Cardamom, Coriander, Jasmine.

Negative attitude about sexuality: Bergamot, Orange, Patchouli, Sandalwood, Rose.

Nervous about sexuality: Ylang Ylang, Geranium, Sandalwood, Jasmine.

Poor social skills: Geranium, Chamomile German or Roman, Lavender, Ylang Ylang.

Unable to appreciate the miracle of life: Orange, Jasmine, Rose, Sandalwood.

Low self-esteem: Juniper, Sandalwood, Ylang Ylang.

Lack of passion, excitement: Jasmine, Sandalwood, Coriander, Patchouli.

Frigidity: Jasmine, Rose, Ylang Ylang, Patchouli, Sandalwood.

Congested Energy
Sexual addiction: Rose, Lavender, Tea Tree.

Strong emotions, mood swings: Lavender, Dill, Vetiver, Geranium, Rosewood.

Too sensitive: Sandalwood, Vetiver, Ylang Ylang.

Emotionally dependent: Rose, Jasmine, Ylang Ylang.

Obsessive attachment: Lavender, Dill, Sandalwood, Rose.

Second Energy Center Blends

<u>A. To encourage sensuality:</u>
Second Center Mist A
6 drops Cardamom
4 drops Jasmine
Mix in 4 ounces of purified water in mister bottle. Shake well before each use.

Second Center Anointing Oil A
2 drops Cardamom
1 drop Jasmine
1 tablespoon jojoba
Mix well together and store in a small glass bottle with a cap.

B. To support safe, loving, and authentic sensuality:
Second Center Mist B
5 drops Rose
5 drops Sandalwood
Mix in 4 ounces of purified water in mister bottle. Shake well before each use.

Second Center Anointing Oil B
2 drops Sandalwood
1 drop Rose
1 tablespoon jojoba
Mix well together and store in a small glass bottle with a cap.

C. To promote sensual joy:
Second Center Mist C
6 drops Orange
3 drops Sandalwood
1 drop Ylang Ylang
Mix in 4 ounces of purified water in mister bottle. Shake well before each use.

Second Center Anointing Oil C
1 drop Orange
1 drop Sandalwood
1 drop Ylang Ylang
1 tablespoon jojoba
Mix well together and store in a small glass bottle with a cap.

D. To calm and balance the emotions:
Second Center Mist D
4 drops Chamomile German or Roman
2 drops Geranium
4 drops Lavender
Mix in 4 ounces of purified water in mister bottle. Shake well before each use.

Second Center Anointing Oil D
1 drop Chamomile German or Roman
1 drop Geranium
1 drop Lavender

1 tablespoon jojoba
Mix well together and store in a small glass bottle with a cap.

E. To promote positive relationships:
Second Center Mist E
4 drops Bergamot
4 drops Orange
2 drops Rosemary
Mix in 4 ounces of purified water in mister bottle. Shake well before each use.

Second Center Anointing Oil E
1 drop Bergamot
1 drop Orange
1 drop Rosemary
1 tablespoon jojoba
Mix well together and store in a small glass bottle with a cap.

Third (Solar Plexus) Energy Center
Essential Oils
Basil: Promotes self-esteem, personal integrity, enthusiasm, and assertiveness.
*Black Pepper: Helps to strengthen personal power. Promotes courage and stamina.
Cedarwood: Promotes confidence, fortitude, and will power.
Chamomile German or Roman: Promotes patience and calm acceptance of our own limitations.
*Clove: Promotes courage, action, and achievement.
Cypress: Promotes confidence and patience, especially during times of change.
*Fennel: Protects against negativity. Promotes courage, confidence, reliability, and assertiveness.
*Ginger: Promotes courage, confidence, and a sense of freedom.
Grapefruit: Promotes confidence, optimism, and spontaneity.
Lavender: Balances personal power.
Lemon: Helps to bring clarity and optimism to personal goals.
Marjoram: Promotes courage, confidence, and personal integrity.
Orange: Promotes an optimistic state of mind.
*Palmarosa: Promotes self-acceptance and personal growth.

*Peppermint: Promotes self-esteem, ethics, and integrity. Helps to overcome feelings of inferiority. Helps to discover personal gifts and strengths.

*Petitgrain: Promotes self-esteem and self-confidence. Encourages trust in self and others. Promotes optimistic attitude.

*Pine: Promotes self-confidence, perseverance, and strength of will.

*Rosemary: Promotes self-confidence and action. Helps to strengthen will power.

*Tea Tree: Promotes confidence, energy, and personal integrity. Helps to strengthen will power.

*Thyme: Promotes self-confidence, personal strength, and courage. Helps to motivate.

Common Imbalances

Constricted Energy

Low energy: Tea Tree, Rosemary, Clove, Pine, Thyme, Lavender.

Inner discontent: Orange, Basil, Fennel, Peppermint, Petitgrain.

Low self-esteem: Rosemary, Basil, Cedarwood, Fennel, Ginger, Palmarosa, Thyme, Petitgrain.

Weak willed: Cypress, Tea Tree, Thyme, Ginger, Cedarwood, Black Pepper.

Easily upset: Peppermint, Black Pepper, Cypress, Orange, Petitgrain, Fennel.

Easily discouraged: Orange, Peppermint, Cypress, Petitgrain, Pine, Tea Tree, Lemon.

Inhibited emotional expression: Marjoram, Ginger, Basil, Clove, Peppermint, Thyme.

Easily stressed in challenging situations: Cedarwood, Basil, Chamomile German or Roman

Unreliable: Basil, Clove, Fennel, Lavender, Peppermint, Tea Tree.

Congested Energy

Manipulative and controlling: Cedarwood, Cypress, Lavender, Peppermint.

Desire to be powerful: Petitgrain, Cedarwood, Basil, Chamomile German or Roman, Lavender.

Unable to relax: Lavender, Chamomile German or Roman, Cedarwood.

Always needs to be right: Lavender, Basil, Chamomile German or Roman, Cedarwood.

Temper outbursts: Chamomile German or Roman, Lavender, Cedarwood, Orange.
Stubborn: Cypress, Lavender, Lemon.
Arrogant: Petitgrain, Basil, Lavender, Petitgrain.
Hyperactive: Chamomile German or Roman, Lavender, Cedarwood.

Third Energy Center Blends

A. To increase self-esteem and confidence:
Third Center Mist A
4 drops Rosemary
4 drops Petitgrain
2 drops Peppermint
Mix in 4 ounces of purified water in mister bottle. Shake well before each use.

Third Center Anointing Oil A
1 drop Rosemary
1 drop Petitgrain
1 drop Peppermint
1 tablespoon jojoba
Mix well together and store in a small glass bottle with a cap.

B. To clear away negative energy or energy blockages:
Third Center Mist B
5 drops Lavender
5 drops Lemon
Mix in 4 ounces of purified water in mister bottle. Shake well before each use.

Third Center Anointing Oil B
1 drop Lavender
2 drops Lemon
1 tablespoon jojoba
Mix well together and store in a small glass bottle with a cap.

C. To release negativity from the past and promote a healthy, self-esteem:

Third Center Mist C
4 drops Orange
3 drops Chamomile German or Roman
2 drops Ginger
Mix in 4 ounces of purified water in mister bottle. Shake well before each use.

Third Center Anointing Oil C
1 drop Orange
1 drop Chamomile German or Roman
1 drop Ginger
1 tablespoon jojoba
Mix well together and store in a small glass bottle with a cap.

D. To feel more energetic:
Third Center Mist D
4 drops Rosemary
4 drops Pine
2 drops Tea Tree
Mix in 4 ounces of purified water in mister bottle. Shake well before each use.

Third Center Anointing Oil D
1 drop Rosemary
1 drop Pine
1 drop Tea Tree
1 tablespoon jojoba
Mix well together and store in a small glass bottle with a cap.

E. To support being more reliable:
Third Center Mist E
4 drops Basil
3 drops Fennel
3 drops Peppermint
Mix in 4 ounces of purified water in mister bottle. Shake well before each use.

Third Center Anointing Oil E
1 drop Basil
1 drop Fennel

1 drop Peppermint
1 tablespoon jojoba
Mix well together and store in a small glass bottle with a cap.

Fourth (Heart) Energy Center
Essential Oils

*Bergamot: Opens the Heart center and allows love and joy to radiate. Eases and comforts wounds of the heart, especially grief. Increases compassion for others' suffering.

Frankincense: Inspires and promotes compassion and service to others.

Geranium: Helps to open our hearts to give and receive nurturing love.

*Helichrysum: Promotes compassion and patience for others and oneself.

Jasmine: Warms and opens the heart. Promotes joy. Helps us to realize our heart's desire.

*Lavender: Calms, comforts, and stabilizes the heart. Promotes compassion, forgiveness, and acceptance.

*Mandarin: Uplifts the heart. Helps a wounded heart to joyfully engage in life.

*Marjoram: Warms the heart. Helps us to accept emotional loss and change. Promotes sincerity and ability to give.

*Melissa: Promotes unconditional love and cheerfulness. Comforts. Eases emotional blocks from grief and shock. Promotes peace and acceptance.

*Neroli: Promotes love and a sense of peace. Eases grief and sorrow.

Orange: Promotes joyful love and cheerfulness. Uplifts a heavy heart.

Patchouli: Helps to open and warm the heart. Strengthens the capacity to care for others.

Petitgrain: Uplifts the heart. Promotes a faith in the power of love.

Pine: Helps to replenish the heart. Promotes generosity.

*Rose: Promotes love, compassion, hope, acceptance, and patience for self and others. Comforts and eases heartaches, especially when the heart is wounded by grief.

Rosemary: Promotes joyful love. Encourages us to help others.

Rosewood: Warms, calms, and comforts the heart. Helps to ease heartaches, especially from childhood.

Sandalwood: Warms the heart and promotes trust.

Vetiver: Helps to calm and strengthen the heart. Helps to protect the compassionate heart.

Ylang Ylang: Integrates passion and peace. Warms and softens a "hard" heart. Promotes the capacity for joy.

Common Imbalances
Constricted Energy
Anti-social: Bergamot, Melissa, Rose, Patchouli, Ylang Ylang, Jasmine.
Disappointed when love is not returned: Rose, Lavender, Neroli, Petitgrain, Melissa.
Unable to receive love: Bergamot, Jasmine, Geranium, Patchouli.
Intolerant of others: Ylang Ylang, Bergamot, Frankincense, Geranium, Helichrysum, Lavender, Patchouli, Rose.
Fear of emotional intimacy: Bergamot, Rose, Jasmine, Lavender, Vetiver, Geranium, Mandarin, Sandalwood, Ylang Ylang.
Overly sensitive: Lavender, Sandalwood, Geranium, Mandarin, Vetiver.
Depressed: Bergamot, Jasmine, Lavender, Mandarin, Marjoram, Melissa, Pine, Rosewood, Neroli, Orange, Ylang Ylang.
Cold and indifferent: Bergamot, Frankincense, Geranium, Mandarin, Orange, Patchouli, Rosewood, Ylang Ylang, Jasmine, Rose, Sandalwood.

Congested Energy
Co-dependent: Geranium, Lavender, Petitgrain, Pine, Vetiver.
Demanding: Bergamot, Geranium, Helichrysum, Marjoram, Rose, Rosemary, Ylang Ylang.
Jealous: Bergamot, Rose, Geranium, Jasmine, Lavender, Marjoram, Patchouli, Pine, Ylang Ylang.
Over-attachment: Geranium, Lavender, Petitgrain, Pine, Vetiver.
Gives too much of oneself: Lavender, Geranium, Pine, Vetiver.

Fourth Energy Center Blends

A. To help heal a wounded heart:
Fourth Center Mist A
7 drops Bergamot
3 drops Rose
Mix in 4 ounces of purified water in mister bottle. Shake well before each use.
Fourth Center Anointing Oil A
2 drops Bergamot

1 drop Rose
1 tablespoon jojoba
Mix well together and store in a small glass bottle with a cap.

B. To support the heart during times of difficult change:
Fourth Center Mist B
4 drops Lavender
4 drops Marjoram
2 drops Vetiver
Mix in 4 ounces of purified water in mister bottle. Shake well before each use.

Fourth Center Anointing Oil B
1 drop Lavender
1 drop Marjoram
1 drop Vetiver
1 tablespoon jojoba
Mix well together and store in a small glass bottle with a cap.

C. To encourage trust in the wisdom of the heart:
Fourth Center Mist C
5 drops Sandalwood
5 drops Petitgrain
Mix in 4 ounces of purified water in mister bottle. Shake well before each use.

Fourth Center Anointing Oil C
2 drops Sandalwood
1 drop Petitgrain
1 tablespoon jojoba
Mix well together and store in a small glass bottle with a cap.

D. To relieve fear of emotional intimacy:
Fourth Center Mist D
4 drops Bergamot
4 drops Sandalwood
2 drops Rose
Mix in 4 ounces of purified water in mister bottle. Shake well before each use.

Fourth Center Anointing Oil D
1 drop Bergamot
1 drop Sandalwood
1 drop Rose
1 tablespoon jojoba
Mix well together and store in a small glass bottle with a cap.

E. To ease intolerance of others:
Fourth Center Mist E
6 drops Frankincense
2 drops Geranium
2 drops Patchouli (or Lavender)
Mix in 4 ounces of purified water in mister bottle. Shake well before each use.

Fourth Center Anointing Oil E
1 drop Frankincense
1 drop Geranium
1 drop Patchloui (or Lavender)
1 tablespoon jojoba
Mix well together and store in a small glass bottle with a cap.

Fifth (Throat) Energy Center

Essential Oils

Basil: Promotes clear, positive communication.
Bergamot: Supports the ability to express compassion and love. Encourages laughter.
Cardamom: Promotes caring verbal communication.
*Chamomile German: Supports calm and gentle speaking of our emotions and truths.
*Chamomile Roman: Supports calm and gentle speaking of our emotions and spiritual truths.
Cypress: Supports our ability to listen.
Geranium: Increases capacity for intimate communication.
Jasmine: Promotes creative expression.
*Lavender: Promotes wise speaking and listening.
Lemon: Promotes focus and clarity in verbal communication.
Neroli: Promotes compassionate communication. Enhances creative expression.

Orange: Clears energy blocks that interfere with ability to communicate (speaking and listening). Supports joyful, verbal communication.
Patchouli: Promotes creative and artistic expression.
Peppermint: Promotes clarity and vitality in communication.
*Petitgrain: Promotes expressiveness and positive communication.
Rose: Promotes wise compassion in verbal communication.
Sandalwood: Promotes harmonious verbal communication.
Tea Tree: Promotes ability to listen and understand different perspectives.
Thyme: Promotes courage to communicate at difficult times.
Ylang Ylang: Promotes calm, warm, and joyful verbal communication.

Common Imbalances
Constricted Energy
Fear of speaking: Chamomile German or Roman, Orange, Thyme, Ylang Ylang.
Weak voice: Chamomile German or Roman, Basil, Peppermint, Petitgrain, Thyme.
Inability to express deep feelings or true self: Chamomile German or Roman, Geranium, Rose, Bergamot, Geranium, Orange, Thyme.

Congested Energy
Speaks harshly: Chamomile German or Roman, Bergamot, Lavender, Neroli, Orange, Rose, Sandalwood, Ylang Ylang.
Talks too much: Chamomile German or Roman, Cypress, Lavender.
Inability to listen: Cypress, Geranium, Lavender, Orange.

Fifth Energy Center Blends

A. To develop effective communication to support close relationships:

Fifth Center Mist A
4 drops Chamomile Roman
4 drops Orange
2 drops Geranium
Mix in 4 ounces of purified water in mister bottle. Shake well before each use.

Fifth Center Anointing Oil A
1 drop Chamomile German
1 drop Orange
1 drop Geranium
1 tablespoon jojoba
Mix well together and store in a small glass bottle with a cap.

B. To communicate one's spiritual truth:
Fifth Center Mist B
5 drops Chamomile Roman
5 drops Rose
Mix in 4 ounces of purified water in mister bottle. Shake well before each use.

Fifth Center Anointing Oil B
2 drops Chamomile Roman
1 drop Rose
1 tablespoon jojoba
Mix well together and store in a small glass bottle with a cap.

C. To promote creative expression:
Fifth Center Mist C
5 drops Jasmine
4 drops Neroli
1 drop Patchouli
Mix in 4 ounces of purified water in mister bottle. Shake well before each use.

Fifth Center Anointing Oil C
1 drop Jasmine
1 drop Neroli
1 drop Patchouli
1 tablespoon jojoba
Mix well together and store in a small glass bottle with a cap.

D. To ease fear of speaking:
Fifth Center Mist D
5 drops Orange
4 drops Chamomile German or Roman
1 drop Thyme

Mix in 4 ounces of purified water in mister bottle. Shake well before each use.

Fifth Center Anointing Oil D
1 drop Orange
1 drop Chamomile German or Roman
1 drop Thyme
1 tablespoon jojoba
Mix well together and store in a small glass bottle with a cap.

E. To promote ability to listen:
Fifth Center Mist E
4 drops Lavender
4 drops Orange
2 drops Cypress
Mix in 4 ounces of purified water in mister bottle. Shake well before each use.

Fifth Center Anointing Oil E
1 drop Lavender
1 drop Orange
1 drop Cypress
1 tablespoon jojoba
Mix well together and store in a small glass bottle with a cap.

Sixth (Brow, Third Eye) Energy Center
Essential Oils
*Anise: Clears away old thought forms. Promotes intuition.
*Basil: Clears the mind. Helps to strengthen the ability to concentrate. Improves ability to calmly make decisions.
*Bay Laurel: Helps to clear mental blocks. Opens the mind to new thoughts and perspectives.
*Benzoin: Steadies and focuses the mind. Helps to bring buried thoughts to consciousness.
Bergamot: Calms and clears the mind. Promotes positive thoughts.
*Cedarwood: Helps to clear and steady the mind. Promotes a strong, calm, positive state of mind. Encourages dreaming.
*Clary Sage: Increases dreaming. Inspires. Supports intuition.
*Elemi: Opens our minds to mystical experiences.

*Eucalyptus: Inspires. Clarifies thoughts and perceptions. Promotes positive thoughts and ability to concentrate.

*Fir: Promotes mental clarity and intuition.

Frankincense: Quiets and clarifies the mind. Promotes introspection, inspiration, and wisdom.

*Grapefruit: Promotes intuition, mental clarity, and alertness. Refreshes the mind and inspires.

Jasmine: Enhances intuition and creative thinking. Inspires.

Juniper: Helps to clear mental stagnation and negativity. Clarifies thoughts. Protects our thoughts from negative influences.

*Lemon: Promotes objectivity, concentration, and mental vitality. Uplifts and clarifies the mind.

*Lemongrass: Promotes mental clarity and flexibility. Supports intuition.

Marjoram: Quiets the mind. Helps to recall memories.

*Peppermint: Stimulates the conscious mind. Promotes clear perception, awareness, and understanding. Inspires and encourages insights. Helps ability to concentrate. Promotes dreaming.

Rose: Promotes wisdom, purity of thought, and intuition. Encourages a sense of mental freedom.

*Rosemary: Energizes and clears the mind. Enhances memory. Promotes clear thoughts, insights, and understanding. Protects the mind from negative influences.

Sandalwood: Quiets the mind. Promotes insights and wisdom.

*Spruce: Helps to develop intuition. Brings objectivity and clarity to the intuitive mind. Encourages new insights.

Common Imbalances

Constricted Energy

Out of touch with reality: Rosemary, Basil, Cedarwood, Grapefruit, Peppermint.

No inner life: Sandalwood, Elemi, Frankincense, Rose.

Poor memory: Rosemary, Basil, Benzoin, Lemon, Marjoram, Peppermint.

Forgetfulness: Rosemary, Basil, Benzoin, Lemon, Marjoram, Peppermint.

Confusion: Basil, Bay Laurel, Cedarwood, Eucalyptus, Fir, Grapefruit, Lemon, Lemongrass, Peppermint, Rosemary.

Congested Energy
Too intellectual: Bay Laurel, Clary Sage, Elemi, Frankincense, Jasmine, Rose.
Intellectual arrogance: Cedarwood, Sandalwood, Frankincense.
Rejects spirituality: Anise, Bay Laurel, Elemi, Juniper, Frankincense, Rose, Sandalwood.
Difficulty concentrating: Basil, Bay Laurel, Cedarwood, Eucalyptus, Fir, Grapefruit, Lemon, Lemongrass, Peppermint, Rosemary.
Nightmares: Frankincense, Bergamot, Cedarwood, Juniper, Rose, Sandalwood.

Sixth Energy Center Blends

A. To promote mental objectivity:
Sixth Center Mist A
5 drops Lemon
3 drops Basil
2 drops Rosemary
Mix in 4 ounces of purified water in mister bottle. Shake well before each use.

Sixth Center Anointing Oil A
1 drop Lemon
1 drop Basil
1 drop Rosemary
1 tablespoon jojoba
Mix well together and store in a small glass bottle with a cap.

B. To support the development of intuition:
Sixth Center Mist B
5 drops Clary Sage
3 drops Jasmine
2 drops Grapefruit.
Mix in 4 ounces of purified water in mister bottle. Shake well before each use.

Sixth Center Anointing Oil B
1 drop Clary Sage
1 drop Jasmine

1 drop Grapefruit
1 tablespoon jojoba
Mix well together and store in a small glass bottle with a cap.

C. To clear and refresh the mind:
Sixth Center Mist C
4 drops Bay Laurel
4 drops Grapefruit
2 drops Rosemary
Mix in 4 ounces of purified water in mister bottle. Shake well before each use.

Sixth Center Anointing Oil C
1 drop Bay Laurel
1 drop Grapefruit
1 drop Rosemary
1 tablespoon jojoba
Mix well together and store in a small glass bottle with a cap.

D. To help improve memory:
Sixth Center Mist D
4 drops Rosemary
4 drops Marjoram
2 drops Peppermint
Mix in 4 ounces of purified water in mister bottle. Shake well before each use.

Sixth Center Anointing Oil D
1 drop Rosemary
1 drop Marjoram
1 drop Peppermint
1 tablespoon jojoba
Mix well together and store in a small glass bottle with a cap.

E. To promote dreaming:
Sixth Center Mist E
6 drops Clary Sage
2 Cedarwood
2 drops Peppermint

Mix in 4 ounces of purified water in mister bottle. Shake well before each use.

Sixth Center Anointing Oil E
1 drop Clary Sage
1 drop Cedarwood
1 drop Peppermint
1 tablespoon jojoba
Mix well together and store in a small glass bottle with a cap.

Seventh (Crown) Energy Center
Essential Oils
*Angelica: Connects us with angelic guidance. Helps to align us with our higher selves.
Basil: Strengthens the sense of spiritual purpose.
Bergamot: Helps to strengthen the connection to Divine love and compassion.
Cedarwood: Promotes a sense of spiritual certainty. Helps to strengthen the connection with the Divine.
Chamomile German: Promotes understanding of spirituality, helping to clear spiritual confusion.
*Elemi: Balances spiritual practices with worldly responsibilities.
Eucalyptus: Promotes a clear connection to spirituality and a sense of oneness.
Fir: Encourages spiritual energy to move through all the energy centers.
*Frankincense: Focuses and strengthens spiritual consciousness and aspirations. Helps us to know our spiritual purpose. Supports our knowing that we are deeply accepted and loved by the Divine. Helps us to heal spiritual wounds.
Jasmine: Heightens spiritual awareness. Helps to connect us with the angelic realm.
Lavender: Helps to integrate spirituality into everyday life. Promotes spiritual growth.
Mandarin: Promotes spiritual joy and tranquility.
Marjoram: Helps to deepen faith during difficult times.
*Myrrh: Helps to strengthen spirituality. Promotes spiritual calmness.
Neroli: Promotes direct communication with the spiritual realm. Helps connect us to angels and to feel guided.

Orange: Represents the joyous light of heaven. Promotes spiritual trust and strengthens a spiritual connection.

Rose: Promotes a close, loving, complete, and devoted spiritual connection. Attracts the angelic realm.

Rosemary: Helps us to remember our spiritual path and dedication. Inspires faith.

*Rosewood: Gently open us to spirituality, as we are ready.

*Sandalwood: Encourages states of higher consciousness, spiritual development, and a sense of spiritual abundance.

Common Imbalances
Constricted Energy
Apathetic: Basil, Cedarwood, Fir, Frankincense, Lavender, Myrrh, Rosemary

Feelings of isolation and separateness: Bergamot, Eucalyptus, Frankincense, Jasmine, Neroli, Orange, Rose.

Lack of purpose: Basil, Cedarwood, Fir, Lavender, Myrrh, Eucalyptus, Rosemary.

Fear of death: Angelica, Bergamot, Cedarwood, Frankincense, Marjoram, Neroli, Orange, Sandalwood.

Congested Energy
Spiritual addiction: Chamomile German, Elemi, Lavender, Rosemary, Sandalwood.

Spiritual Confusion: Cedarwood, Chamomile German, Elemi, Frankincense, Jasmine, Lavender, Orange, Rosemary.

Disassociation with body: Chamomile German, Elemi, Fir, Lavender, Myrrh, Sandalwood.

Seventh Energy Center Blends

A. To bring all the energy centers into balance and unify them with the Divine:
Seventh Center Mist A
4 drops Frankincense
4 drops Lavender
2 drops Fir
Mix in 4 ounces of purified water in mister bottle. Shake well before each use.

Seventh Center Anointing Oil A
1 drop Frankincense
1 drop Lavender
1 drop Fir
1 tablespoon jojoba
Mix well together and store in a small glass bottle with a cap.

B. To open us to spiritual guidance and love from the angelic realm:
Seventh Center Mist B
4 drops Rose
4 drops Mandarin
2 drops Neroli
Mix in 4 ounces of purified water in mister bottle. Shake well before each use.

Seventh Center Anointing Oil B
1 drop Rose
1 drop Mandarin
1 drop Neroli
1 tablespoon jojoba
Mix well together and store in a small glass bottle with a cap.

C. To integrate spirituality into our daily lives:
Seventh Center Mist C
6 drops Lavender
2 drops Elemi
2 drops Myrrh
Mix in 4 ounces of purified water in mister bottle. Shake well before each use.

Seventh Center Anointing Oil C
1 drop Lavender
1 drop Elemi
1 drop Myrrh
1 tablespoon jojoba
Mix well together and store in a small glass bottle with a cap.

D. To develop a sense of spiritual purpose:
Seventh Center Mist D
4 drops Frankincense

4 drops Chamomile German
2 drops Basil
Mix in 4 ounces of purified water in mister bottle. Shake well before each use.

Seventh Center Anointing Oil D
1 drop Frankincense
1 drop Chamomile German
1 drop Basil
1 tablespoon jojoba
Mix well together and store in a small glass bottle with a cap.

E. To ease a fear of death:
Seventh Center Mist E
4 drops Bergamot
4 drops Orange
2 drops Frankincense
Mix in 4 ounces of purified water in mister bottle. Shake well before each use.

Seventh Center Anointing Oil E
1 drop Bergamot
1 drop Orange
1 drop Frankincense
1 tablespoon jojoba
Mix well together and store in a small glass bottle with a cap.

Hands Energy Centers
Essential Oils
Basil: Supports being of service to others.
*Bergamot: Supports the ability to give positive, healing energy.
Black Pepper: Promotes the ability to give and receive without judgment.
*Cardamom: Helps us respond to someone in need.
*Chamomile German or Roman: Helps to receive and give healing energy.
Elemi: Promotes positive giving and receiving.
Fir: Clears energy blocks to promote healthy giving and receiving.
Frankincense: Promotes the ability to send compassion through touch.

*Geranium: Promotes gentle, nurturing healing energy.
*Helichrysum: Promotes healing energy.
Jasmine: Enhances creative and artistic development.
Juniper: Protects us from absorbing negative energy when touching someone else.
*Lavender: Promotes healing energy and sensitivity to it.
Neroli: Helps to balance giving and receiving.
Nutmeg: Enhances creative expression.
Orange: Promotes joyous healing energy.
*Rose: Connects the hands to the heart. Promotes compassionate healing energy.
*Rosewood: Promotes ability to send healing energy.
Sandalwood: Promotes calming, healing energy.
Spruce: Promotes cleansing energy.

Common Imbalances
Constricted Energy
Difficulty giving and receiving: Chamomile German or Roman, Lavender, Elemi, Fir, Neroli.
Low healing energy: Bergamot, Lavender, Helichrysum, Sandalwood.
Disconnected from self and others: Frankincense, Geranium, Rose, Orange, Bergamot.
Blocked creativity: Nutmeg, Jasmine.

Congested Energy
Poor personal boundaries: Juniper, Fir, Bergamot.
Physical and/or psychological exhaustion: Juniper, Elemi, Neroli.
Resentment/bitterness: Lavender, Rose, Orange, Black Pepper.

Hands Energy Centers Blends

A. To support being of service to others:
Hands Centers Mist A
5 drops Bergamot
5 drops Basil
Mix in 4 ounces of purified water in mister bottle. Shake well before each use.

Hands Centers Anointing Oil A
2 drops Bergamot
1 drop Basil
1 tablespoon jojoba
Mix well together and store in a small glass bottle with a cap.

B. To balance giving and receiving:
Hands Centers Mist B
6 drops Chamomile German or Roman
2 drops Elemi
2 drops Fir
Mix in 4 ounces of purified water in mister bottle. Shake well before each use.

Hands Centers Anointing Oil B
1 drop Chamomile German or Roman
1 drop Elemi
1 drop Fir
1 tablespoon jojoba
Mix well together and store in a small glass bottle with a cap.

C. To promote compassionate touch:
Hands Centers Mist C
4 drops Lavender
3 drops Rose
3 drops Frankincense
Mix in 4 ounces of purified water in mister bottle. Shake well before each use.

Hands Centers Anointing Oil C
1 drop Lavender
1 drop Rose
1 drop Frankincense
1 tablespoon jojoba
Mix well together and store in a small glass bottle with a cap.

D. To promote ability to send healing energy:
Hands Centers Mist D
5 drops Rosewood
5 drops Lavender

Mix in 4 ounces of purified water in mister bottle. Shake well before each use.

Hands Centers Anointing Oil D
2 drops Rosewood
1 drop Lavender
1 tablespoon jojoba
Mix well together and store in a small glass bottle with a cap.

E. To develop/build up healing energy:
Hands Centers Mist E
4 drops Bergamot
3 drops Helichrysum
3 drops Lavender
Mix in 4 ounces of purified water in mister bottle. Shake well before each use.

Hands Centers Anointing Oil E
1 drop Bergamot
1 drop Helichrysum
1 drop Lavender
1 tablespoon jojoba
Mix well together and store in a small glass bottle with a cap.

Feet Energy Centers
Essential Oils
*Benzoin: Grounds. Encourages walking gently on the earth.
Black Pepper: Grounds and strengthens the body's energy.101
Cardamom: Grounds and reassures.
*Cedarwood: Promotes grounded spirituality.
Cypress: Grounds and stabilizes. Helpful during times of change.
Fir: Grounds. Promotes stability and flexibility.
*Frankincense: Grounds. Connects our spirituality with the earth.
Ginger: Grounds and rejuvenates.
Helichrysum: Grounds and stabilizes.
Lavender: Grounds healing energy to support and strengthen.
Marjoram: Grounds and comforts.
*Myrrh: Grounds the lower energy centers.
*Oakmoss: Grounds. Helps "spiritual" people to value earthly life.

*Patchouli: Grounds. Helps to connect us with the earth's energy.
Peppermint: Grounds and energizes.
Rose: Grounds and stabilizes.
*Rosewood: Grounds. Supports a healing process.
*Sandalwood: Grounds and stabilizes. Promotes grounded spirituality.
Tea Tree: Grounds and energizes.
*Vetiver: Grounds, balances, and protects.

Common Imbalances
Constricted Energy
Ungrounded: Vetiver, Sandalwood, Cardamom, Helichrysum, Patchouli.
Emotionally unstable: Cardamom, Rose, Fir, Marjoram, Sandalwood.
Mentally confused: Cypress, Rose, Peppermint, Cedarwood, Sandalwood.
Depressed: Cypress, Peppermint, Rosewood, Sandalwood, Vetiver, Tea Tree.
Rejection of/fear of the earth plane: Benzoin, Cardamom, Cedarwood, Fir, Marjoram, Oakmoss, Patchouli, Sandalwood.
Disconnected from life force: Black Pepper, Cardamom, Fir, Ginger, Lavender, Oakmoss, Patchouli, Tea Tree, Vetiver.

Congested Energy
Physical addiction: Black Pepper, Peppermint, Fir, Helichrysum, Marjoram, Rosewood, Cypress.
Psychological addiction: Cardamom, Cypress, Fir, Helichrysum, Peppermint, Rosewood, Sandalwood, Rose.
Disconnected from spirituality: Cedarwood, Frankincense, Sandalwood.
Apathetic: Ginger, Peppermint, Tea Tree.

Feet Energy Centers Blends

A. To promote a sense of being grounded:
Feet Centers Mist A
4 drops Sandalwood
4 drops Cardamom
2 drops Vetiver

Mix in 4 ounces of purified water in mister bottle. Shake well before each use.

Feet Centers Anointing Oil A
1 drop Sandalwood
1 drop Cardamom
1 drop Vetiver
1 tablespoon jojoba
Mix well together and store in a small glass bottle with a cap.

B. To help stabilize the emotions:
Feet Centers Mist B
4 drops Fir
4 drops Rose
2 drops Patchouli
Mix in 4 ounces of purified water in mister bottle. Shake well before each use.

Feet Centers Anointing Oil B
1 drop Fir
1 drop Rose
1 drop Patchouli
1 tablespoon jojoba
Mix well together and store in a small glass bottle with a cap.

C. To help relieve mental confusion:
Feet Centers Mist C
4 drops Cedarwood
4 drops Sandalwood
2 drops Peppermint
Mix in 4 ounces of purified water in mister bottle. Shake well before each use.

Feet Centers Anointing Oil C
1 drop Cedarwood
1 drop Sandalwood
1 drop Peppermint
1 tablespoon jojoba
Mix well together and store in a small glass bottle with a cap.

D. To help embrace earthy life:
Feet Centers Mist D
5 drops Cardamom
4 drops Marjoram
1 drop Patchouli
Mix in 4 ounces of purified water in mister bottle. Shake well before each use.

Feet Centers Anointing Oil D
1 drop Cardamom
1 drop Marjoram
1 drop Patchouli
1 tablespoon jojoba
Mix well together and store in a small glass bottle with a cap.

E. To help connect with spirituality:
Feet Centers Mist E
4 drops Cedarwood
3 drops Frankincense
3 drops Sandalwood
Mix in 4 ounces of purified water in mister bottle. Shake well before each use.

Feet Centers Anointing Oil E
1 drop Cedarwood
1 drop Frankincense
1 drop Sandalwood
1 tablespoon jojoba
Mix well together and store in a small glass bottle with a cap.

Chapter 5: Helping Ourselves

"Energy. We want it, and we are drawn to people who radiate it. When we have it, we feel great, and when we don't, we feel as though we're missing out on life. How can we be stewards of our vital energy, cultivating it, and manifesting more when we need it?"

—William Collinge, *Subtle Energy*

Cultivating and having vital energy helps us to feel good and function well. It's the "get up and go" that enriches our life and makes it possible for us to do what we want. It also enables us to give to those around us. This vital energy is gathered, supported, and maintained by taking care of ourselves—practicing self-care. It involves many things, such as nourishing and exercising both our bodies and minds, reducing and managing stress, tending to our meaningful relationships, embracing our spirituality, and living a healthy, positive lifestyle in all ways possible.

The energy we have is not static. It is an ever-changing, dynamic, and evolving process, which can be increased and strengthened by self-care, and depleted by a lack of it. It is important to acknowledge that no one does this perfectly. As you go through the Self-care Questionnaire and The Four Dimensions of Well-Being, notice the areas that you would like to improve and then do the best you can to accomplish them. Be kind and forgiving to yourself as you go through the process of making positive changes. *This is the essence of self-care.* The goal of being perfect is unrealistic and not possible. Be gentle, and again, do all that you can.

Self-care Questionnaire

Self-care is the foundation of a nurturing, supportive relationship with yourself. When you take care of yourself, you acknowledge the requirements and rewards of being your own true friend. You tend to the child within you and fulfill, as best you can, the needs of your body/mind/spirit, such as play, work, sleep, rest, companionship, purpose, love, beauty, and spirituality.

Subtle energy therapy emphasizes the need for self-care so that you have enough energy to be able to draw and receive healing energy into your physical and subtle bodies. This is necessary to support good health and well-being. It also enables you to be able to send healing energy to others.

Many people find it a challenge to be as kind to themselves as they are to others. It is not uncommon for people to find it hard to *receive*. The reasons for this are many and may be revealed to you after completing this questionnaire. Before you begin working with subtle energy therapy, for yourself or for others, examine your thoughts, beliefs, and feelings about *receiving* and the idea of *self-care*. Answer the following questions. Take time to do it thoughtfully and thoroughly, and then reflect upon your responses to gain understanding.

"Receiving" and You

1. Generally, am I comfortable or uncomfortable about receiving help from others?
2. What are the situations in which I feel comfortable? What makes these situations comfortable?
3. Are there particular people from whom I am comfortable receiving help? What makes me feel comfortable with these people?
4. What are the situations in which I feel uncomfortable receiving help? What makes them uncomfortable?
5. Are there particular people from whom I am uncomfortable receiving help? What makes me feel uncomfortable with these people?
6. What does selfishness mean to me?
7. Can I remember a time in which I behaved selfishly? If so, what was going on with me and/or the other person (people) that resulted in my behavior?
8. How would I describe the difference between selfishness and healthy self-care?
9. Has there been a situation in which receiving help from someone felt selfish? If so, what made me feel selfish?
10. Can I remember a time in which my refusing help from others felt like an act of selfishness? If so, what was going on with me and/or the other person (people) that made me feel selfish?

"Self-care" and You

1. What does self-care mean to me? How do I feel about it?
2. What am I currently doing to take care of myself in each of the following areas?
Exercising:
Eating healthfully:

Getting enough sleep:
Resting:
Working:
Learning:
Creating:
Playing:
Tending to my relationships:
Maintaining a social network:
Spending time with others:
Living in a nurturing home environment:
Having/bringing beauty into my life:
Being responsible with finances:
Being in service to others:
Cultivating a spiritual practice:
Are there any other areas of self-care not mentioned here that are important for you?

3. Are things missing in my self-care practice? If so, what are they? What prevents me from including them? What could help me include them?

4. Who supports me in my efforts to take care of myself? How do they support me? How does this affect me? How do I respond to their support?

5. Who is not supportive of me in my efforts to take care of myself? How do they not support me? How does this affect me? How do I respond to their lack of support?

6. If I could take one step to improve my self-care, what would it be? What would help me take that step? When could I realistically take that step? Notice if there are other steps you might be willing and able to take following this first step.

7. How will you honor and celebrate your choices for improving your self-care?

The Four Dimensions of Well-being

The level and strength of your energy depends on the vitality of the four dimensions that determine your health and well-being: physical, mental, emotional, and spiritual. The description of each dimension below is followed by a few questions. Answer these questions, ponder your responses, and reflect on their meaning in relationship to the level of energy you have and changes you may want to make in your life.

1. Physical Well-being (Diet, Exercise, Rest, Sleep)

<u>Diet</u>. Primary to physical health is eating healthy, nourishing food—as the rule and not the exception. We all have different nutritional needs based on our biochemical individuality, and we have different nutritional needs at different times of our lives.

Nutritional advise from health care practitioners and nutritionists is inconsistent and changes over time. This makes it difficult to follow guidelines but, in fact, as more research is done, more information is available. It makes sense that, as more is known, creating and maintaining good health through nutrition may change. So, it is important to learn about healthy eating and revisit how you eat periodically. There is an abundance of information on the Internet. As well, consider seeing a nutritionist to help you design an eating program that is right for you.

Ask yourself:
Am I eating the best food for my health?
How does my current diet make me feel?
Do I have the energy I need to do what I want to do?
Am I eating consciously?
Do I have enough variety in my diet?
Do I enjoy my food?
What can I do to improve my eating habits?
Should I see a nutritionist?

<u>Exercise</u>. Regular exercise is also primary to physical health. The human body is designed for action and movement. It wears faster from disuse than it does from use and operates better with more movement and work than less. Being physically fit is a part of good health.

There are exercise programs for everyone. Ideally, they would include aerobics, strengthening, and stretching. Regular aerobic exercise strengthens the heart muscle, increases circulation, makes bones less brittle, improves mental health, improves lung function, and makes the body more resilient and resistant to disease. Strengthening makes you stronger, promotes bone health and muscle mass, and promotes better body mechanics. Stretching reduces muscle tension, increases range of motion, promotes muscular coordination, and increases circulation. Consider working with a physical fitness professional to design a program that is right for you.

Ask yourself:
What are my forms of exercise?
Do I include aerobics, strengthening, and stretching?
How often do I exercise?
Do I need to make more time for exercise? If so, how can I do this?
Do I enjoy exercising? If not, what can be done to make it more pleasurable?
How can I improve my exercise program?
Should I see a fitness professional?

Rest. In the plant and animal world, we see many examples of the natural rhythm of activity followed by rest. Bears hunt and eat, and then hibernate. A puppy plays hard, and then collapses and sleeps. A plant that flowers in summer is dormant during winter. Nature teaches us that a balance of rest and activity supports strength, growth, and creativity.

Wayne Muller, author of *Sabbath: Remembering the Sacred Rhythm of Rest and Delight*, says, "Because we do not rest, we lose our way. We miss the compass points that show us where to go. We lose the nourishment that gives us succor. We miss the quiet that gives us wisdom." Take some time each day for pleasurable rest such as taking a nap, reading a book, watching a little television, or listening to music. Discover what is restful and restorative for you and give yourself permission to enjoy it.

Ask yourself:
Do I partake in pleasurable rest everyday? If not, what prevents me?
What form of rest is best for me?
What form of rest do I enjoy?
What benefits do I receive from resting everyday?
How can I make rest a part of my daily routine?

Sleep. Sleep repairs and rejuvenates your body, mind, and spirit. If you are getting enough sleep, you wake up without an alarm, feeling refreshed, revitalized, and ready for the day.

To avoid energy depletion, you need an optimum amount of sleep every night. This is believed to be between seven and eight hours, however, this can vary with the seasons or during times of illness or emotional stress. Getting enough sleep on a regular basis is what is required for optimum renewal.

Ask yourself:

How many hours of sleep do I regularly get every night?

If I am not getting enough sleep, what can I do to get more? (Should I go to bed earlier? Can I take a short nap during the day?)

If I am not getting quality sleep, what can I do to improve it?

Would it be helpful to speak with my health care provider about the duration and quality of my sleep?

2. Mental Well-being (Work, Study and Create, Play)

Work. Whether it is a paid job, volunteer assignments, or parenting children, your work in the world is one of the most important and time-consuming parts of your life. It contributes greatly to your self-definition, sense of purpose, and self-esteem.

Love of work is rewarding, satisfying, and builds energy. However, overwork, unrewarding work, and unpleasant work can be depleting. It is particularly important after a rough day at work to take care of yourself to rebuild your energy. It may mean having some alone time or it may mean being with a dear friend. It may mean taking a short nap, taking a bath, treating yourself to a dinner out, watching a movie, reading, or just doing nothing. When workdays are good, that alone will help build up energy reserves.

Ask yourself:

Is my work enjoyable most of the time?

What ways, if any, can make my work situation better?

Do I value what I am doing?

In what ways is my work meaningful to me?

How is my energy before, during, and after work?

Study and Create. Activities that engage and challenge your mind strengthens your mental and creative capacities. Choose exercises for both sides of your brain—the logical left and the creative right. To improve and energize your logical mind, take classes, go to interesting educational lectures, learn how to do something new, do a crossword puzzle, or engage in stimulating conversation. For your creative mind, explore the arts, listen to music, draw, write, or go to the theater. Practice keeping your mental activities (left and right brains) in balance because when they are unbalanced, your mental as well as physical energy can be depleted.

Ask yourself:

What do I do regularly to challenge my logical mind?

What do I do regularly to cultivate my creative mind?

Which do I enjoy more?

Are my mental activities in balance? If not, what can I do to improve the balance?

Play. Play came naturally to us when we were children, but as we grew older, we had more responsibilities and available playtime was less. Play is important for everyone, of all ages, to energize and free the body, mind, and spirit. Play helps us to have some unstructured time, free of responsibilities and commitments. Play has no agenda or goals. It is for the experience itself. It is simply, yet profoundly, just for fun. Play adds joy and laughter to our life, relieves stress, and helps us to feel young and energized.

Play is personal. It is whatever is fun for you and whatever makes you smile and laugh and feel good. This could be playing a game of softball with friends, playing a game of pee wee golf, going to a waterslide park, spending time with a favorite hobby, going to the beach, playing with your pets, going for a bike ride, singing, or dancing to your favorite music. Play promotes joy, increases your energy and creativity, and reduces stress.

Ask yourself:

What do I enjoy as play?

What makes me laugh?

How often do I play?

How can I bring more playfulness into my life?

3. Emotional Well-being

Your emotional life is made from an accumulation of past and present life experiences—primarily with yourself and other people but also with work, hobbies, and personal goals. Emotions are powerful and complex and can be both constructive and destructive to your state of well-being. For example, love, compassion, and joy expand your energy. Hate, jealousy, and fear deplete your energy.

Tending to your emotions involves cultivating a loving relationship with yourself, forming a social network, nurturing your relationships, and spending time doing the activities that positively support your self-esteem. It involves learning how to recognize and acknowledge your true feelings, and then being able to move through them and express them in a healthy way. It involves integrating the "darker" aspects of yourself so that you can become a more whole and complete emotional being. It may also involve making necessary changes in your life and maybe with some of your relationships. If you need help with this process, there are competent professionals that can assist you. As you learn to support and experience emotional well-being, your energy builds and strengthens.

Ask yourself:
What brings me a sense of emotional fulfillment?
What emotions are easy/easier for me to feel? Why?
What emotions do I resist feeling? Why?
Which relationships make me feel good?
Which relationships drain me?
What relationships support me in being emotionally alive?
Am I spending enough time with the people I love?
How can I improve my relationships?
What activities do I do that make me feel good?
What activities do I do that drain me?
What activities support me being emotionally alive?
How can I incorporate into my life more positive, uplifting people and activities?
What experiences in my life do I value?
What unhealthy habits would I like to stop?

4. Spiritual Well-being

Everybody has a spiritual dimension. It is a part of being human. Spirituality is, at heart, the place where we connect to that which is greater than ourselves. For some, this may mean embracing God in our life or having a meditation practice. For others, it may mean hiking in nature, or being involved with charities that serve mankind.

Worldly success is often measured by our vocation, family life, wealth, or fame. Yet, there are many outwardly successful people who feel empty and wonder why they are not happy. This is an example, from a subtle energy standpoint, of a depleted Seventh (Crown) energy center, our center for spirituality.

Traditionally, spirituality has been nurtured by church communities, meditation groups, nature ceremonies, or through sacred dance and song. However, there are other profound, non-religious ways to strengthen your sense of spirituality, such as working in a garden or being inspired by great art, music, or literature. For many, giving and receiving energy healing, and working with essential oils is a spiritual experience.

As your spiritual nature grows, everything you do and experience can strengthen your well-being in this dimension. Washing the dishes can become a prayer, gardening can be an act of worship, and doing the laundry can be an act of contemplation and gratitude. Along with the practices and ceremonies we set aside as sacred, there grows an illuminating sense that even the most mundane act can be holy. As the Seventh energy center draws spiritual light into your being, your entire energy field is infused with brilliance, and you can give—to yourself and others—without depletion.

Ask yourself:
What is "spirituality" for me?
What is sacred to me?
Do I feel connected to something greater than myself?
How would I describe my relationship to spirituality?
What in my life supports my spiritual well-being?
Do I have a spiritual practice? If not, would I like to have one? If so, is there anything that I would like to add to my spiritual practice?

A Self-care Exercise: 20 Things I Would Be Doing If...

Write down a list, entitled, "20 Things I Would Be Doing if I was Taking Care of Myself."

This is an exercise that gives you a big picture of the changes you may want to make in your life to better take care of yourself. You might include things such as "walk every morning" or "improve my diet" or "visit my neighbor more." Think about all the elements of your life, such as those mentioned in the "The Four Dimensions of Well-being." Take your time and make it authentic and meaningful.

When you are finished, look at the list and choose ONE thing that seems possible for you to accomplish right now and do it. Focus on it. It may be your top priority, or it may not be. (Give yourself permission to try something else if you decide this first choice is not workable for you at this time.)

The time it takes to establish a new habit varies with every individual. It may take you a week or longer. On average, it takes two months for a new habit to be securely in place. Give yourself permission to take as long as you need. When you feel you are ready to move on, choose another item from your list.

If it is a big goal, such as "eat a healthy diet," don't let it overwhelm you. Break it down further into small, simple steps that you will work with one at a time. Be sure to make these baby steps specific, such as "I will eat carrot sticks with my lunch," rather than, "I will eat more vegetables." Or "I will take a multi-vitamin with breakfast," rather than, "I will start taking supplements." The simpler the steps, the easier they are to commit to and accomplish. This technique fosters a wonderful sense of success.

There is an interesting thing that can happen when you begin making the positive changes you want in your life. Sometimes, when good habits are established in one area, it affects other areas, almost without you being aware of it. So, when you look at your original "20 Things," after you have accomplished one, some of your other goals on the list may have changed or may no longer be a goal for you. Adjust your list accordingly. It will be a living process that reflects where you are currently on your self-care journey.

Remember, not judging yourself is a part of self-care. Do the best you can to incorporate healthy habits. Find what works for you at the moment. Appreciate every bit of improvement you make. A little counts for a lot because every time you practice your new habit, you are telling your body/mind/spirit, "I care for you!"

Stress: A Part of Life

Stress is an unavoidable part of a full life and managing it well can make life a little easier. It is also an important part of taking care of yourself. So significant, stress reduction and management could be considered #5 in the "The Four Dimensions of Well-Being."

Stress can contribute to your evolving personal growth and development and it can cause depletion and health problems. Stress, as defined in Webster's Dictionary, is "mental or physical pressure, challenge, or strain." Eustress, or "good stress," is the positive response to experiences and events that are challenging but are found fulfilling, nevertheless. Eustress may come from having a welcomed new baby or landing a dream job. It may also come from complex situations, such as physical or emotional therapy that involves some discomfort but leads to deep healing. Although eustress is positive, it can still put a strain on you, and if you are dealing with several stresses at once, such as a new baby, moving to a new home, and changes at work, it can be overwhelming and require special support.

Dis-stress, or "negative stress," is the negative response to experiences and events that are physically or emotionally difficult. It may be from going through a divorce, dealing with a health crisis, losing your job, or having relationship problems. One of the most common forms of stress today is chronic, low-level stress, which includes factors such as a long commute, noise pollution, not having enough money to make ends meet, or not having enough time to get everything done. This on-going stress can wear us down and cause physical and mental health issues.

The body produces the stress hormones, cortisol and adrenaline, when it is under pressure. Nature developed this as a defense mechanism known as "fight or flight." When the "danger" is over, the production of these hormones should stop. But in the case of chronic stress, the production continues at a low, on-going level. This is linked to depressed immune function, inflammation in the body, gastrointestinal problems, increased physical pain, interference with sex hormones, heart disease, and increased storage of fat.

Unfortunately, all the information about how we must reduce our stress can also contribute to stress!

Stress Reduction and Stress Management

There are two steps to dealing with the stress in your life: stress reduction and stress management. Stress reduction involves looking at your life and seeing what can be done to reduce the negative stress in it. Stress management is what you do after you have made those changes, to maintain a level of stress that is manageable and healthy for you.

Stress Reduction Questionnaire

Ask yourself:

What aspects of my life cause me negative stress?

What aspects of my life, that cause negative stress, are non-negotiable to change? Why?

What aspects of my life, that cause negative stress, am I able to consider changing? Why? How would you be able to change these things? (For example, if bad news in the morning newspaper depresses your outlook for the day, you can stop reading the newspaper and look for another way to find out about the news that is important to you.)

Can the stressor be broken down into aspects I can work with one at a time?

Is there a way for me to get more rest to help counteract stress, such as going to bed earlier, sleeping in a bit later, or taking a ten-minute nap during the day?

Is there someone I could sit down with who could help me look at my life, from an outside perspective, as to what might be helpful and possible to think about changing?

After answering these questions and gaining insight to your particular situation, make a list of the things that are causing negative stress in your life that you are ready and willing to change. Choose one and do it. When you have successfully changed the situation, choose another, and so on, until you feel the stress in your life has been reduced and is now more manageable.

Now you need to explore how you can best deal with the stress that remains and shore up your ability to cope with it to become more stress resilient. There are many techniques to do this. They may include exercise, dietary guidelines, breathing exercises, guided imagery, meditation, more sleep, supportive relationships, relaxation techniques, and/or a spiritual practice. It will require taking some time to review the variety of techniques, and then deciding what is realistic for you and what feels like a fit for you and your circumstances. It could mean making changes in your life such as scheduling time for yourself, learning to say "no," and knowing your limitations. Reflect on managing stress in terms of your physical body, your emotions, your intellect, and your spirit.

Stress Management Questionnaire

Ask yourself:

Do I have support in my life for stress management? If so, what is it? If not, how might I get some support?

Do I need to prioritize my stressors? If so, which one(s) will I first address? Why?

How might I best approach managing my stress?

What stress management techniques will I first try? Why?

Can I develop an initial stress management program to try that realistically addresses the various (physical, emotional, intellectual, and spiritual) stresses in my life? What makes this program realistic?

How will I check if this program is helping me? What will I be watching for? Are there people in my life that can help me check how this program is working?

What are my goals for this stress management program?

Three Breathing Exercises

To help you get started, we offer here three different breathing exercises. They can be useful to help you to relax and achieve a calm state of mind. Breathing is something that you can control and manage. Practiced regularly, these exercises can help with stress-related problems. (There are many more breathing exercises that can be found on the Internet. Dr. Andrew Weil, a Harvard-trained medical doctor who is renowned for his work in integrative medicine, is a strong supporter of using breathing exercises to counteract stress.)

1. Relaxing Breath. Sit comfortably with your back straight. Exhale completely through your mouth. Close your mouth and inhale through your nose for a count of three. Hold your breath for a count of five. Exhale through your mouth to a count of six. Repeat slowly and gently three more times.

2. Relaxation Response Breath. Sit comfortably with your back straight. Exhale, make an audible sigh, drop your shoulders, and relax your entire body. Inhale gently and completely. Repeat three more times.

3. Breath Meditation. This exercise is designed to help you relieve stress by breathing and identifying 1) what you need to let go of and 2) what you want to bring in, such as letting go of ill feelings associated with a relationship issue and bringing in forgiveness. To begin, identify in your mind the stressor and the feelings associated with it. Then take

a slow, gentle breath in and as you exhale imagine them being released from your body, mind, and spirit. Then inhale slowly and gently again as you imagine filling yourself with what you need to be whole, healthy, and at peace. Repeat this for ten breaths, breathing slowly and evenly and taking an extra breath in between if you need to. (You can also do this exercise by imagining when you exhale that you are releasing out through the bottom of your feet and bringing in through the top of your head.)

Aromatherapy

Aromatherapy and subtle energy techniques may also be useful for you in your stress management program. They can shift your body/mind/spirit into being both relaxed (for anxious stress) and gently uplifted (for lethargic stress) in a way that can assist you in your daily life.

Many essential oils are excellent for stress relief. Some of our favorites are Bergamot (relaxes yet uplifts), Chamomile Roman (relaxes), Lavender (relaxes and uplifts), Neroli (relaxes and uplifts), Clary Sage (relaxes and uplifts), Marjoram (relaxes), Frankincense (relaxes), and Orange (uplifts).

These essential oils can be used in a variety of ways. While using them in any of the following ways, hold the intention of the purpose for which you are using them as described in Chapter 2.

1. Inhalation: Put a drop or two on a tissue and inhale the aroma through your nose. Pause and repeat inhalation.

2. Massage: Make a massage oil by mixing twelve drops of the essential oil(s) in one ounce of fragrance-free lotion or carrier oil such as fractionated coconut oil. While breathing in the aroma, massage your hands, feet, neck, and shoulders. You may also want to schedule a massage with a professional and have then use your aromatherapy massage oil. Massage is an excellent way to relax the body and relieve stress. (This is a stronger dilution than is normally used for subtle aromatherapy in order to accommodate a physical relaxation response.)

3. Bath: Fill your tub with warm water. Immerse yourself. Mix together one teaspoon of carrier oil and eight drops of essential oil. Add to the water and stir and gently massage your skin while you breathe in the aroma.

4. Body Mister: Add twenty drops of essential oil(s) into a four-ounce misting bottle filled with water. Shake well before each use. Avoid getting the mist into your eyes. Breathe in the aroma.

5. Simple Hold. This subtle energy technique is described in the list below, #16, and can be used for stress relief by holding the part of your body in which you feel the stress.

Emotions Associated with the Energy Centers

Our sense of good health, wholeness, and aliveness depends, in part, on being able to truly feel all our emotions, and then appropriately respond to them in a balanced, healthy way. In Chapter 2, many aspects of each energy center are described. There, you learned about the emotions that are associated with each center, when it is in balanced and imbalanced states. Here, we provide more information about emotions along with questions that are designed to help you gain insight into *your* emotions and how they may be processed.

In our lives, on a daily basis, we experience both expanding, pleasant feelings and contracting, unpleasant ones. Emotional states can affect the energy centers to create balance or imbalance. Emotional balance refers to the capacity to both feel and allow the movement or flow of any given emotional experience, to complete its process. This makes us "whole" as human beings. Imbalance refers to emotions losing their movement and becoming "stuck." This occurs because we, in some way, interfere with the process and range of emotions. This imbalance occurs primarily in three ways.

1. We reject certain emotions. Typically, this means pushing away or becoming numb to unpleasant or challenging emotions such as grief, anger, or fear. Unprocessed grief can become depression, anger can become bitterness, and if fear is immobilized, one may become fearful about life itself. Some of us might even push away and reject pleasant emotions because previous experiences have caused us to distrust them.

2. We cling to certain emotions. This means trying to hold on to feelings such as joy, a sense of peace, or love because they are pleasant. Clinging can falsify their sincere presence. All emotions come and go, though they may have a presence that is underlying. One emotion may be replaced by another at any given moment. If we become attached to joy, we may avoid feeling sad and may drive away those around us who

are experiencing life's challenges. We might identify with peace and then refuse to deal with conflict and challenging situations. Those who cling to love can regress to co-dependence. Some of us might even cling to painful feelings because we are familiar with them.

3. We try to take charge of the length of time of an emotional process. Emotions are a *feeling* process; they are rarely a *cognitive* process. When we use our mental capacity to force or "pretend" that we no longer feel a certain way, it may not align with or allow for the authentic timing of the emotional process.

Please be aware that unpleasant and challenging emotions are not "bad" or "wrong," though they, indeed, may be uncomfortable and difficult. They are, instead, like all our emotions, signals. Fear alerts us to situations that may be dangerous. Guilt and shame can provide the impetus to change our behavior or make amends. Grief is the natural response to loss and a part of the heart's healing process.

As you go through the following questions, make notes of any relevant thoughts you may have. Reflect upon you answers. Use this for insights into your feelings so you may come to understanding. Ask yourself:

1. Does my fear immobilize me, or am I able to use it to create more safety, security, and trust? 2. Does my guilt or shame paralyze me into believing that I am unworthy, or assist me in determining to be a better and more loving human being?

3. Does my grief permanently shut down my heart or help me realize the preciousness of life—the gifts of this tender, fleeting existence?

4. Does my sense of helplessness prevent me from pursuing the life I was created to live?

5. Does my selfishness help me listen to myself so I can hear others?

6. Does becoming aware of my close-mindedness help me discern what I truly believe and help me to be willing to examine those beliefs?

7. Does pain about my life and the situation of the world close me off from spiritual sustenance, or does it encourage me to find ways to practice hope?

8. Does greed cause me to shut off from others or does it help me look at what I really want?

9. Does feeling disconnected cause me to abandon myself or encourage me to seek ways to serve others?

Assessing Your Energy Centers

As you have learned, your energy centers reflect your current state—physically, mentally, emotionally, and spiritually. As a part of self-care, you can pay attention to the state of your energy centers and then take steps to restore harmony, balance, and strength when needed.

How do you know if your energy centers are out of balance? You may cognitively or intuitively know simply by what is happening in your life. For example, if you have recently experienced a loss or are grieving, your Fourth (Heart) center will likely be out of balance. If you are in the throes of finals at school, it is likely your Sixth (Brow) center will be out of balance. If you are struggling in a relationship, your Second (Sacral) energy center could be out of balance. In addition, you might be experiencing physical symptoms such as a headache or stomachache which would indicate an imbalance in the centers that govern these areas.

Here, we offer two additional ways to assess your energy centers 1) by taking and interpreting the Energy Center Questionnaire and 2) by having a friend help you "read" your energy centers with a pendulum.

Hopefully, when all this information comes together, you will understand the current state of each of your energy centers and can work towards balancing them by working with the information in Chapter 4 and the exercises below in "Balancing Your Energy Centers and Subtle Bodies."

Energy Center Questionnaire

Answering yes to four or more of the questions associated with a specific energy center may indicate an imbalance. Because energy centers are in flux, you should take this questionnaire periodically. If your life is stable, you may want to check in with it every three months or so. If you are in crisis or there are lots of changes going on, you may want to check it as often as it is helpful—maybe once a week.

First (Root, Base)

Do you feel disassociated from your body?
Are you overweight?
Are you underweight?
Do you have a weak physical constitution?
Does life on earth feel like a burden?

Are you fearful?
Are you disorganized?
Are you possessive and/or materialistic?
Are you worried about financial security?
Are you accident-prone?

Second (Sacral)

Do you suppress your sexual desires?
Do you have a negative attitude about sex?
Are you obsessed with sexual thoughts or feelings?
Does sexuality make you nervous?
Are you emotionally dependent or detached?
Do you have emotional swings?
Do you lack passion or excitement about life?
Does your creativity feel blocked?
Do you feel guilty?
Are you having problems in relationships?
Are you afraid of making a commitment?

Third (Solar Plexus)

Do you have low energy?
Do you have low self-esteem?
Are you weak willed?
Are you easily upset or discouraged?
Do you feel ashamed of who you are?
Are you unreliable?
Are you manipulative and controlling?
Are you unable to relax?
Do you have temper outbursts?
Are you stubborn?
Are you prone to digestive problems?
Do you always like to be in control?
Are you afraid of rejection?
Do you try too hard to please others?

Fourth (Heart)

Are you anti-social?
Are you intolerant of others?
Do you have a fear of intimacy?
Are you overly sensitive?

Are you depressed?
Are you grieving?
Are you indifferent?
Do you have a jealous nature?
Do you have difficulty forgiving?
Do you have difficulty breathing?
Do you take care of others but not yourself?

Fifth (Throat)

Do you have a fear of speaking?
Do you have a weak voice?
Are you unable to express your true feelings?
Are you shy or withdrawn?
Do you speak harshly to others?
Do you talk too much?
Do you tell lies?
Are you selfish?
Are you unable to listen to others?
Do you frequently have a sore throat?
Do you feel you have nothing worthwhile to say?
Do you clench your jaw or grind your teeth?
Do you often feel rushed—that you don't have enough time?

Sixth (Brow, Third Eye)

Are you out of touch with reality?
Do you have a poor memory?
Are you forgetful?
Do you feel confused?
Do you have impaired vision?
Do you have difficulty concentrating?
Do you have nightmares?
Do you often misunderstand situations?
Do you have frequent headaches?
Are you over-analytical?
Are you close minded?
Do you doubt your intuition?

Seventh (Crown)

Are your apathetic?
Do you feel lonely or isolated?

Do you feel you have no purpose in life?

Are you afraid of dying?

Does life seem senseless?

Are you over-attached to your belongings or relationships?

Do you have an addictive relationship with spirituality?

Do you search for answers outside yourself?

Hands

Is it difficult for you to receive?

Do you feel uncomfortable or unsafe when others want to give to you?

Do you have trouble identifying what you need/want?

Is it difficult for you to give?

Do you distrust others?

Are you feeling empty, with little or nothing left to offer?

Are you experiencing compassion-fatigue? (Check your Heart center as well.)

Do you feel depleted from too much activity and outflow of energy?

Do you want to cling to people/situations/experiences?

Are you pushing away what nurtures you?

Feet

Do you feel ungrounded?

Do you feel disconnected from your body and the messages your body may be sending you?

Do you feel unstable in your life, relationships, and/or relationship with yourself?

Do you feel physically weak?

Do you feel weighted down?

Do you feel a lack of energy?

Do you have trouble concentrating?

Are you afraid of losing your sense of self and your own boundaries?

Are you resistant to vigorous exercise?

After you have completed the questionnaire, you will likely have a good idea as to which of your energy centers may be out of balance. To further assess them, you may want to check them with a pendulum (see below, "Using a Pendulum"). You will need someone that is familiar with using a pendulum to help you.

Once you are aware of which energy center or centers are currently out of balance (remember, they are always in flux), there are techniques and essential oils that can help bring them back into balance. These are discussed at length in Chapter 4 and more information follows below in "Balancing Your Energy Centers and Subtle Bodies."

Using a Pendulum

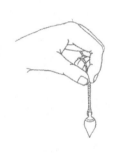

To assess your energy centers with a pendulum, you will need a friend to help you. Your friend will need to know how to use a pendulum. (If they do not, instructions for using a pendulum are readily available on the Internet.)

A pendulum consists of a weight secured at the end of a chain or string. The chain needs to be long enough (six inches or more) to allow the weight to swing freely. You may purchase a pendulum made of materials such as brass or crystal, but it is just as effective to make one with a piece of thin string and a small weight, such as a button.

A pendulum can be a useful tool to test the current state of the energy centers. The swing of a pendulum demonstrates energy flow, showing in its movement if the energy center is constricted (too little energy—indicated by a small swing), congested (too much energy—indicated by a large swing), or balanced (a healthy amount of energy—a medium swing).

A healthy energy center sets the pendulum spinning clockwise in a circle. If out-of-balance, the pendulum might be still, move in the other direction (counter-clockwise), or swing in an odd shape such as an oval or flat-line. Finally, a balanced energy center system would be indicated by the pendulum swinging at relatively the same size and shape for each center.

To pendulum-test the energy centers, the person being tested should be lying down. The person who is testing holds the chain or string of the pendulum so the weight is about three inches away from the body of the person lying down. The pendulum is held over one of their energy centers. (Usually, the First energy center is tested first and then the Second, and so on up to the Seventh.) The tester's arm and hand must be still and wait for the pendulum to move. It will begin to respond to the center's energy field, moving in the circular direction, size, and shape of the energy center, giving you an indication of its current state.

It is interesting to note, that if the energy centers were assessed the next day, they may demonstrate differently. This is because they are constantly changing and reflecting the current state of the person.

If you are using a pendulum, it takes a little practice to feel confident about what the pendulum is demonstrating. However, remember that it is only a tool, and you may intuitively feel that the energy center is in a different state than what the pendulum is indicating. In this case, use your best judgment, remembering that your intention is for balancing and healing.

Balancing Your Energy Centers and Subtle Bodies

Following are a variety of different exercises that you can do to help balance and strengthen your energy centers and subtle bodies. At any given time, choose the exercise that feels right to you.

1. Four Dimensions

Review all your answers from the section, "The Four Dimensions of Well-being." Make a list of things you would like to work on. Pick one and write down how you are going to introduce this change into your life. Allow yourself two months in which to accomplish it.

At the end of each week, assess your progress. If you have been successful, determine what contributed to your success. If not, determine what prevented it from happening. Was your goal realistic? If so, what will you do so that it can be accomplished next week? If not, how can you change your goal to make it realistic? Repeat this process at the end of each week.

Keep in mind that perfectionism drains energy. Do the best you can, be realistic about your goals and start slowly. It usually takes about two months for a new habit to become solidly entrenched in your lifestyle.

When you are ready, pick another item from your list, and go through the same process. Notice how the positive changes have affected other areas of your life, and look forward to enjoying a new level of well-being. As you build vitality, your well-being in all dimensions is strengthened.

2. Subtle Energy Therapy

Giving or receiving subtle energy therapy helps to balance and strengthen the energy centers and subtle bodies. Because the subtle anatomy is an interconnected web, subtle energy therapy for any energy center will help to further balance and harmonize the entire system. This will assist any aspect of the subtle anatomy that might be impacted, even minutely, by the imbalance being addressed. Schedule a time to give or receive a subtle energy therapy session.

3. Taking Time / Making Time

Thomas Merton, an American Catholic writer and mystic, said, "To allow ourselves to be carried away by a multitude of conflicting concerns, to surrender to too many demands, to commit oneself to too many projects, to want to help everyone in everything, is to succumb to suffering." "Suffering" seems like a strong word to use but Merton believes that when we are busy all the time, even busy with good things, the frenzy "kills the root of inner wisdom." Even though we are trying to do good work, if we are frantic, worn-out, or overextended, we will unintentionally create imbalance.

Many peoples' lives are very busy and the desire to take care of oneself is often thwarted by not being able to find the time or the motivation. Authentic self-care may require a re-shuffling of priorities, cutting back on responsibilities, and striving to simply do less.

Completing the following exercise will help you prioritize how you spend your time, making more time available for self-care and things that build your energy. Do this exercise as often as necessary to keep your life on track with being only as busy as is healthy for you.

A. Make a list of all the things you spend your time doing.
B. Separate this list into 3 columns, assigning each their priority:
1) *Top priorities.* These are the most important things to you that need to be accomplished. It might be shopping for food, working, cooking, exercising at the gym, or paying bills.
2) *Second priorities.* These are important but not as important as top priority items. They might be doing the laundry, cleaning the house, writing letters, reading, or shopping for clothes.

3) *Lowest priorities.* These are things that are not so important, but some of the things on this list can move up to second or top priority if put off too long, such as bathing the dog or mowing the lawn.

C. Go through each column and assign to each item how often it is done—daily, weekly, monthly.

D. Review the lowest priorities. Is there anything you would be willing to change? For example, could you spend less time on social media, perhaps posting less frequently? Could you read just the Sunday paper and not the daily? Could you plant a garden that requires less care?

E. Review the second priorities. Is there anything that can be moved to lowest priority or be done in an easier way?

F. Review top priorities. Is there anything that can be moved to second priority or be done in an easier way?

G. Place your name above each of the three columns. Review each column. What self-care practices are in your top priority column per day, week, and month? Your second priority column? Your lowest priority column? If there aren't any or just a few, it's time to insert self-care activities into all three lists that support your well-being on a daily, weekly, and monthly basis. Such as, adding a daily walk, a weekly dinner out, and a monthly massage.

4. Warm Bath or Shower

Taking a warm bath or shower can relax as well as revitalize your body, mind, and spirit, depending on the intention and the essential oils used. The process of washing your physical body sends a signal to your subtle anatomy that this is a time of cleansing away all that needs cleansing and no longer needed.

A. Bath. Put one cup of apple cider vinegar or two cups of Epsom salts in a tub of warm water. Stir well. Immerse yourself and remain in the tub for about fifteen minutes while you visualize your subtle anatomy being balanced and nurtured. After the bath, let all the water drain out of the tub while you visualize your body and soul letting go of what it no longer needs. Then rinse yourself thoroughly with warm water to remove any residue. Finish with a cool water rinse, towel dry, dress, and then rest for an hour while sipping a tall glass of room-temperature water.

B. Shower. Take a warm, ten-minute shower. After the shower, while your skin in still wet, put three drops of Cedarwood, Juniper, Rosemary, or Lavender in the palm of one hand, pat your hands together, then quickly and evenly apply to your arms, legs, and torso while you visualize clearing and cleansing. (Do not apply to face or sensitive areas.)

NOTE: Showers and baths are not recommended on the day of receiving subtle energy therapy, so as not to disrupt the newly established energy pattern.

5. Helpful Daydreams

To integrate self-care practices and make healthy changes in your life, a simple and common visualization technique, similar to daydreaming, can assist you in programming yourself.

Get comfortable. You may be sitting or lying down. Close your eyes and take three deep, relaxing breaths. In your imagination, visualize and experience making a change in your life and taking care of yourself in a new way that you would like, such as exercising regularly. See yourself and feel yourself doing it. Watch yourself as if you were on a movie screen and it was reality. Bring in all your senses. What do you see? How do you feel? Are there any sounds that you can hear? Are there any aromas or tastes? Let this experience become as clear and real as possible, knowing that you are now positively programming yourself to incorporate this change. When you have internally practiced and integrated changes in your life in this way, it becomes easier to manifest them outwardly in reality.

This next step is optional. If there is an essential oil that relates to and supports your desired change, you can inhale its aroma during this exercise, and give yourself the suggestion that each time you smell it, it becomes easier and more natural for you to practice your new self-care behavior. (This is a guided imagery technique.) In this way, the essential oil becomes an anchor, and can assist you in making your desired change. Some essential oil suggestions are Bergamot for optimism, Clove for achievement, Helichrysum for patience, Lavender for healing and balance, Frankincense for feeling calm, Eucalyptus for positive thinking, Marjoram for acceptance, Jasmine for creativity, Rosemary for motivation, or Pine for rejuvenation. Review Chapter 3 to find other essential oils that you may want to use.

6. Creating

Creative activities help to balance your subtle anatomy and connect you with the creative life force that is within you. They draw on your imagination and visions. This practice of creating is not about being a good "artist." It is about allowing the original process of creativity to flow through you as you make, invent, form, conceive, discover, and design something that expresses who you are and what you want to express.

Our suggested directive in cultivating and being creative is to allow yourself to play. Make something beautiful that pleases you and that you have fun doing. Experiment creating with mirrors, bells, flowers, fabric, feathers, rocks, shells, or glass. Create a meal of your favorite foods. Write a song and sing it with a tune you create. Pen a creative poem or description of something that you love or makes you feel happy.

The essential oils that especially support creativity are Bay Laurel, Cardamom, Coriander, Geranium, Ginger, Helichrysum, Jasmine, Neroli, Nutmeg, Patchouli, Rose, and Rosewood. They can be used by diffusing, anointing, stroking, or misting, as described in Chapter 4. Remember, that no matter which essential oil you choose to use, use it with the intention of the purpose you desire.

Jasmine, Neroli, Patchouli, Rose, and Rosewood nurture the skin and can be used in a massage oil, body mist, or bath to help promote creativity. Make the massage lotion with eight drops of essential oil in one ounce of fragrance-free lotion. Make a body mist by mixing ten to fifteen drops in a four-ounce misting bottle filled with water. Shake well before each use. Use in a bath by filling the tub with warm water, immersing yourself, then adding eight drops of essential oil to one teaspoon of carrier oil. Stir in the mixture and massage your skin while you inhale the aroma.

7. Nourishment Through the Senses

Our good health and well-being are affected by what our five senses come in contact with during the day and during our lives. Taste, touch, sight, hearing, and smell are all avenues into our psyche and impact us. Ideally, we would live in and see a beautiful, peaceful environment, eat nourishing food, hear lovely sounds, experience beautiful aromas, and spend time with wonderful people. Because, realistically, this is not usually the case, we can do the best we can by making choices that are positive, build vital energy, and support taking care of ourselves. We can choose to fill our living space with beautiful things and things that please us. We can choose to eat a variety of healthy, delicious food. We can choose to listen to music that uplifts our spirits. We can choose to fill our living space with pleasant aromas, and we can choose to spend time with people that make us feel good.

As you review each of the five senses, make a list of the things you can do for each one to improve what is impacting you in your daily life. Think about the eliminating unwanted influences as well as adding welcomed ones.

Tasting: Ayurveda teaches that there are six different tastes, each of which you could encounter every day to stimulate different parts of your brain. They are sweet (such as bread, honey), sour (such as yogurt, lemon), salty (such as pickles, soy sauce), bitter (such as spinach, endive), astringent (such as beans, pomegranate), and pungent (such as pepper, ginger). Eat healthy foods that you like so you have a pleasurable experience. Cultivate your taste to enjoy a variety of tastes and vary what you eat.

Touching: Human beings need to be lovingly touched for good health. Your skin is replete with nerve endings that stimulate and send messages to your brain. Hugs and handholds help you feel connected and provide emotional nourishment. Hug your friends. Hold hands with your sweetheart. Shake hands with new acquaintances. Schedule a massage.

Seeing: What is visually appealing to you? Natural settings such as gardens? Magnificent architecture such as churches? Bright colors or soft colors? Geometric or rounded designs? Serve your eyes a feast. Bring things into your home and workplace that are visually pleasing to you in both color and design. Place things that are meaningful or nostalgic to you, such as pictures of dear friends. Take a walk in a park or garden. Look through books of a favorite artist's work or visit an art museum.

Hearing: Music was an integral part of ancient Egyptian medicine and the Greeks believed that music restored health to both body and soul. It is thought that certain types of music (generally soft and soothing tones) cause the body to release endorphins that can relieve pain and induce relaxation. Music can also be used to energize and uplift. Listen to your favorite music. Visit a church and listen to the choir. Go to a concert of your favorite band.

Interestingly, silence is also therapeutic. Anthropologist Angeles Arien says, that in many indigenous tribes, the healer will ask an ill person, "When did you lose your love of the sweet territory of silence?" Silence is the sound of the Seventh energy center and can be very rejuvenating to experience—a welcome respite from a noisy world. Use earplugs, if possible, when you are exposed to noise that is unsettling for you.

Smelling: As you have learned through aromatherapy, aromas affect you on many levels. When odor molecules enter your nose, they affect the limbic system in the brain, causing physiological and psychological responses. Aromatherapy uses natural aromas from plants to relax, relieve stress and anxiety, ease depression, and energize. Inhale the aromas of your favorite essential oils through your nose. Smell foods that you enjoy. Eliminate unpleasant odors.

8. Being Present

Being present is the capacity to be aware, awake, alert, attuned, open-minded, and openhearted *in the present moment*. It is being aware of and tending to the external world as well as your internal world—with all your senses and your intuition. When you are in the present moment, there is a sense of freedom and peace and it helps to balance all your energy centers. Practicing being *aware* helps develop the ability to be fully present. The following exercise will help you to experience greater awareness.

Awareness Exercise

Sit comfortably. Bring all your attention to where you are at the moment and take a deep breath.

Take notice of all your senses and what they are experiencing. Begin with what you *see* and be aware of it for a few moments. Move on to the other senses, one by one, each for a few moments. Be aware of what you *smell*. Be aware of what you might be *tasting*. Be aware of what you are *hearing*. Lastly, move on to what your body and hands are physically *touching* or being touched by. When you are finished with this last sensation, pull it all together and feel fully present in your body, mind, and spirit, and breathe deeply and gently until you are ready to go move forward with your day.

9. Affirmations

Affirmations are brief, positive intention statements. They are simple, yet powerful, and can help balance your energy centers. They can be said internally or out loud. They can be used whenever you smell or apply essential oil(s). Below are some suggested ones, but, as always, tailor these to suit your needs or create your own.

First (Root)
I am safe.
I am healthy and strong.
I have all that I need.
I experience abundance in my life.
I am grounded and centered.

Second (Sacral)
I celebrate my body and sensuality.
I enjoy my sexuality.
I freely and easily create.
I feel my feelings, and they give me important information about myself and others.
I invite healthy and supportive relationships into my life.
I experience joy in my life.

Third (Solar Plexus)
I appreciate who I am and what I do.
I always hold healthy and appropriate boundaries.
I manifest what I need and want.
I am a person of integrity and courage.
I am confident in my abilities.

Fourth (Heart)
I am love.
I accept and love myself and others.
I am guided by faith and strengthened by hope.
I love my body and my mind.
It is safe for me to open myself to giving and receiving love.

Fifth (Throat)
I speak my truth.
I listen with loving, thoughtful attention.
What I have to say is worthy of being expressed and heard.
I know when to speak and when to be silent.
I have all the time I need.

Sixth (Brow)
My mind is clear and focused.
I trust my intuition.
My mind is open to new ideas, new perspectives.
I discern what is, for me, the truth.
My mind is clear, calm, and infinite.
I am wise.

Seventh (Crown)
I am connected with my spiritual path.
I am filled with the light of spirit/God.
I trust in spirit/God.
I bring spirituality into my daily life.
Each moment is divine.
I love and am loved by spirit/God.

Hands
I am able to give.
I am able to receive.
I discern what I want in my life.
I receive the love of the universe.
I have enough.
I am enough.

Feet
I am connected to the earth.
I am stable and strong.
I am centered in my body/mind/spirit.
I am flexible and responsive.
I am a part of the whole.
All is connected.

10. Positive Actions to Strengthen Your Energy Centers

Following are a few suggestions of things you can do to help strengthen and balance each of your energy centers. Remember, your lifestyle and experiences affect your energy centers.

First (Root, Base): Take care of yourself. Maintain a weight that is healthy for you. Rest, eat well, and exercise. Do work you love.

Develop a conscious relationship with money. Organize. Say an affirmation that you have a positive attitude about life.

Second (Sacral): Give and receive. Create. Play. Do things that you enjoy. Explore joyful sexuality. Say an affirmation that you are comfortable with your feelings.

Third (Solar Plexus): Accomplish a goal. Learn to relax. Be proud of who you are. Express your anger in constructive ways. Be responsible. Say an affirmation that you attract what you want in your life.

Fourth (Heart): Give love and compassion unconditionally. Be sincere. Accept yourself and others. Be patient with yourself and others. Nurture yourself and others. Breathe deeply. Say an affirmation that you are at peace.

Fifth (Throat): Speak the truth. Speak gently. Sing or chant. Express yourself. Listen well. Take time. Say an affirmation that you express yourself freely and creatively.

Sixth (Brow, Third Eye): Visualize. Imagine. Intuit. Study. Reflect. Learn something new. Write down your dreams. Say an affirmation that you have a clear and perceptive mind.

Seventh (Crown): See the Divine in everybody, everywhere. Feel a sense of oneness and a sense of purpose. Cultivate faith. Align yourself with the Divine before you act or speak. Look inside yourself for answers. Say an affirmation that you are one with the universe.

Hands: Practice giving without attachment. Practice 'letting go'. Massage your hands. Visualize that you receive what you want from the Universe. Say an affirmation that you give and receive in a balanced, healthy way.

Feet: Dance. Walk and practice being fully present while you are walking (see #8). Massage your feet. Mentally, take a healthy, firm stand in an area of your life that needs you to be firm and balanced. Say an affirmation that you are grounded and balanced in your life.

11. Energy Workouts

Yoga, qi gong, and tai chi help to balance the energy centers and build vital energy. Classes and instructors can be found on the

Internet. Local community centers often offer classes. Many gyms have now incorporated yoga and other forms of energy workouts.

We also suggest dancing or just moving your body, standing or sitting, as you are able. Find music that generates the type of energy you want for yourself at the time. Do you feel like moving fast or slow or something in between? Whatever it is, allow your body to get into it. Then think about each of your energy centers and visualize each of them in a healthy, balanced state as described in Chapter 2.

12. Tending to an Energy Center

The following exercise is designed to tend to an energy center that you have chosen.

A. Choose an essential oil appropriate for that center. (This information is in Chapter 4.) Place a drop on the palm of one of your hands and then pat your hands together. (If you have sensitive skin, mix the essential oil with a little fragrance-free lotion before applying.) Breathe in the aroma with the intention to create balance and harmony in the chosen energy center.

B. When you are clear about your intention, create an energy ball between your hands, as described in Chapter 2, "Feeling Subtle Energy with Your Hands."

C. Then allow a color to come into that energy ball. Use the color associated with that particular energy center, as described in Chapter 2.

D. Hold the energy ball, now infused with the subtle properties of an essential oil and color, over the energy center that you want to tend to, keeping the intention of balance and healing in your mind. Hold the ball there until you feel you are done.

E. After this process, write down any ideas that may come to you about how you might support the intention of tending to this energy center.

13. Tending Touch

This exercise brings tenderness and healing into your body, mind, and spirit. It uses life-giving breath to support self-care.

A. On a tissue, put a drop or two of an essential oil that you have chosen to use to support your practice of self-care. Inhale the aroma through your nose. Pause and inhale again. There are many essential oils to choose from. Perhaps you now have a favorite. Some of our favorites are Rose, Lavender, Sandalwood, Rosemary, Orange, and Bergamot. (You can read more about these essential oils and others in Chapter 3.)

B. Get into a comfortable position—lying down, sitting, or standing. Gently rest your dominant hand on your heart and your non-dominant hand on your stomach.

C. Gently breathe, as fully as you can, to first fill your stomach and then your lungs. Do this ten times, slowly and completely. While doing this, include an intention, affirmation, or prayer that supports taking care of yourself.

14. Helping Hand

This simple, self-care exercise is from Jin Shin Jitsu, a Japanese system of energy healing that works with your subtle anatomy. According to this system, each finger on your hand is connected to a heart/mind state. Gently holding that finger will bring balance so that there is neither congestion (overstimulation) nor constriction (depletion). It promotes being grounded, relaxed, and energized, accompanied with healthy thoughts and feelings.

The thumb balances the state of worry.
The forefinger balances the state of fear.
The middle finger balances the states of anger and frustration.
The ring finger balances the state of sorrow.
The little finger balances the energy of forcing an issue ("trying to…").

There are two main approaches to working with Helping Hand, focused and general. Choose the one that seems right for you at the time.

A. Focused: For a specific emotion or mental state you want to address, hold that particular finger, with intention, for a minute or until you sense a gentle pulsing in the finger. You can use either hand.

B. General: For a general balancing, you can: 1) Hold each of your ten fingers, with intention, for a minute or until you sense a gentle pulsing in each finger or 2) Hold one of your thumbs for ten minutes. The thumb balances all states. This can be done even when you are not focusing on it. Set your intention and then just hold your thumb. You can do this while meditating, watching TV, at an office meeting, or in any situation in which holding your thumb would not be obtrusive.

At the end of the hold(s), slightly shake out your hand and look forward to being more present and able to go about your day and attend to what is needed.

If you would like, you can use essential oils with this exercise. If you are doing a Focused hold, anoint the holding hand and breathe in the aroma with the intention of balancing the particular emotional/mental state. Then, begin the hold. We suggest for the thumb, Jasmine for worry. For the forefinger, Marjoram, Neroli, or Thyme for fear. For the middle finger, Ylang Ylang, Benzoin, or Black Pepper for anger/frustration. For the ring finger, Chamomile German, Myrrh, or Neroli for sorrow. For the little finger, Chamomile German or Roman for forcing an issue.

If you are doing a General hold, anoint both your hands on the palms with Lavender, Geranium, Cedarwood, Clary Sage, or Elemi. Gently pat your hands together. Breathe in the aroma, as you hold the intention of balancing your subtle anatomy. Then, begin the finger holds or thumb hold.

15. Simple Hold

Simple Hold is one of the basic hand positions that is used in subtle energy therapy and is included with other hand positions that are described in Chapter 6: Helping Others. It is the only one that is well suited to use by oneself. Simple Hold is designed to work with specific areas of the body, bringing them into balance so that the body's natural healing ability can unfold.

To do Simple Hold, place your hands on either side of any area of your body that needs attention—side-to-side or front to back. It might be an injury, an ache, or a particular energy center. This position is done with your hands touching your body, but it can be off your body in the energy field for situations that might be uncomfortable to touch. Hold the intention of healing in your mind and visualize a gentle wave of healing energy moving from one hand to the other, passing through the area in need, until the energy flow feels even or continuous, or until you sense that it is finished. If you need to, this position can be done with one hand or one hand on top of the other, to gently send the healing energy until you sense the area is full.

As you practice, you will discover your own way of knowing when the hold is finished. Some people see an image of completion, others sense a tingling in their hands, and others just "know." There is no right or wrong way. In the beginning, you may feel more comfortable holding for a prescribed amount of time, and we would recommend three to five minutes.

If you would like, combine using color with Simple Hold. Visualize an appropriate color (such as blue or lavender for inflammation, red for increasing circulation, green for balancing, orange for yellow for rejuvenating, or pink for love), moving back and forth between your hands—glowing clear, bright, and strong.

If you choose to use essential oils with Simple Hold, they can be chosen four different ways, whichever way feels right to you at the time.

1. Body Parts: Different organs and body parts are associated with and influenced by specific energy centers. (See Chapter 2, as a reference for each energy center, under "Gland association" and "Parts of body influenced.") For example, the thyroid is associated with the Fifth (Throat) energy center. The throat, the mouth, the ears, the neck, and the nose are influenced by it.

Identify the body area in need (such as the stomach), identify the energy center associated with it (the Third), and then choose an essential oil that works with the needs of that energy center (such as Rosemary, Orange, or Lavender). To help you choose the essential oil, we recommend using "The Essential Oils for the Energy Centers" as a reference in Chapter 4. Then use Simple Hold to work with the associated energy center with the intention of benefitting the body part in need.

2. Mental / Emotional Issues: Choose an essential oil that addresses the mental or emotional issue, such as mental fatigue or fear. Other issues might be grief, loneliness, envy, low self-esteem, irritability, sorrow, apathy, confusion, poor memory, or worry. (Chapters 3 and 4 will provide you with the information you need to determine this.) As examples for fear, Orange eases depression and promotes feelings of joy, helping to counteract fear; Cedarwood calms a fearful mind; Ylang Ylang relaxes the body and mind to reduce fear; and Rosemary reduces mental confusion often associated with fear.

Then, work with the energy center that relates to the issue (see Chapter 4 as a reference, under "Working with the Energy Centers"). As examples, grief is related to the Fourth, low self-esteem is related to the Third, and worry is related to the Sixth. You can also work with the place on the body where the symptoms are felt. Most people feel emotional symptoms in the head, throat, chest, and/or stomach. So, if you are working with someone else, you will need to ask where he or she feels the emotion. Fear is often felt in the chest, worry in the head, and grief in the head, throat, heart, and stomach areas.

3. Energy Centers: Common imbalances of each energy center are covered in Chapter 4. Choose an essential oil that meets the appropriate need of the energy center. (Chapter 3, which lists the subtle energy properties of fifty-five different essential oils, will help you with this. Tea Tree helps to energize when depleted; Black Pepper helps to clear energy blocks; Lavender helps to balance and bring in positive energy; Lemon helps to clear and cleanse; and Pine helps to clear away negative energy strengthen energy flow.) Then, work with the energy center itself, placing your hands on the front and back of the body or by using the one-hand method.

4. Physical Symptoms / Physical Locations: Choose the essential oil that assists with the physical symptom, and then work in the area of the symptom. As examples, use Eucalyptus for respiratory congestion with your hands over the lung area; use Peppermint for indigestion with your hand over the stomach area; and use Rosemary for a tired muscle with your hands over that muscle. (Because these physical level uses of essential oils are not addressed in this book, if you are unfamiliar with the physical uses, we recommend using a reference book that has this information. A few suggestions are *Practical Aromatherapy for Self-care* by Joni Keim and *Aromatherapy: A Lifetime Guide to Healing with Essential Oils* by Valerie Gennari Cooksley.

Simple Hold Positions to Help Specific Situations
1. Hands cupped over the eyes: Relieves anxiety, reduces stress, relaxes, and promotes mental clarity.
2. Hands covering the temples: Relieves worry, reduces stress, and promotes calmness and mental clarity.
3. Hands covering the back of the head: Reduces fear and worry, relieves stress, and promotes a sense of well-being.
4. Hands over the throat: Relieves anger, resentment, and frustration, and promotes feelings of security.
5. Hands over the heart: Promotes relaxation, comforts, and reduces stress.
6. Hands over the liver/stomach: Reduces stress and anxiety, relieves frustration, and promotes self-confidence.

7. Hands over the lower stomach: Releases anger and fear and promotes creativity.

8. Hands cupping over the ears: Promotes receptivity to inner and outer information.

9. Hands on the ankles: Releases tension and stress.

10. Hands on the knees: Releases tension and stress, releases challenging emotions, and promotes forgiveness.

11. Hands on the wrists: Releases tension and stress, and promotes creative expression.

12. Hands on elbows: Releases tension and stress, and promotes interaction with one's environment.

13. Hands on the shoulders: Releases tension and stress, and motivates.

Chapter 6: Helping Others

Ethical Responsibility

If you want to offer to give someone a subtle energy therapy session, whether it is a family member, a friend, or a client, you have certain ethical responsibilities. Your task is to create a comfortable and emotionally safe place in which to work; to be in a positive, compassionate state of mind; to be open to the healing energy of the universe; to have the intention of helping, and to establish a respectful, caring relationship with the person.

Remember, when you work with someone with the intention of promoting health and well-being, the healer is *within that person*, the receiver. Your role is to facilitate a process, not to "fix" the receiver or expect a certain outcome. The body/mind wisdom of the receiver will use what you provide in the best way possible. Your intention is to be of the most beneficial service to your receiver. Allow energy and the receiver's innate healing ability to do the rest.

Avoid judging or blaming someone for what they are experiencing. Telling someone they have a headache because they "shouldn't have eaten chocolate" or they "need to release anger" is inappropriate and may be entirely wrong. Shaming the receiver is counter-productive and constricts their energy field. It also does not support the compassionate qualities of *your* Heart center. Accept, without judgment, whatever condition the receiver is in.

Confidentiality is necessary to establish trust between you and the receiver. Never discuss what happens in a subtle energy therapy session with anyone else unless it is a professional supervisor. This even includes not discussing the session with the receiver outside of the session time itself. For example, if your receiver is a friend that you see regularly, recognize that the session is a special and separate occasion. Do not casually refer to it outside of that time unless they choose to discuss it.

Respect the receiver's limits and personal boundaries. People have different comfort levels concerning physical touch and emotional sharing. Not every receiver wants a hug. Not everyone will want to talk in depth about his or her present symptoms, or about themselves. Part of creating an emotionally safe environment for the receiver is to let them know that you recognize and honor their boundaries.

We recommend that a subtle energy therapy session be given with as little dialogue as possible. Pay particular attention to keeping your personal sharing to a minimum. Share, without judgment, only when it will make the receiver know that you understand and can empathize with them. A session is their time to receive. If, however, the receiver feels the need to talk, it may be a part of their healing process. In this case, be a good listener.

Active Listening

If you want to give subtle energy therapy sessions, you must be able to be a good listener—an active listener. It is a great gift to offer your receiver the remarkable experience of being truly and fully heard. For many, it is healing in itself. To be an active listener, listen closely and acknowledge what you hear. Pay attention to the following.

Body language. While someone is talking, if you turn your back to him or her, neglect to make eye contact, or are busy doing something else, you are sending body language signals that you are not paying attention. Instead, situate yourself at a comfortable distance from the receiver, face them, and occasionally make eye contact. Be calm and comfortable. This signals to the receiver that you are present and interested.

Paraphrasing. Occasionally, repeat back to the receiver what you have heard from them. For example, "Let me tell you what I've heard you say, and you can tell me if I am understanding you accurately." This lets the receiver know you are listening and gives them an opportunity to correct any misunderstandings. It can be helpful as well as reassuring.

Ask open-ended questions. Do not assume that you know what the receiver is experiencing with comments such as, "That must be hard for you," or "You must be really angry." In fact, it may not have been hard for them, or they may not have been angry. Instead, ask open-ended questions such as, "How did you feel?" or "What was that like for you?" This allows for a deeper sharing of their experience.

Misplaced empathy. Do not assume you know someone's experience because you had a similar one. Avoid statements such as, "I know exactly what you are going through." Most people resent this comment because, in truth, you do not know—everyone experiences life differently. However, sometimes this type of sharing can be helpful in making the person feel not so alone. "I've had bad sinus headaches, too, and they can be really painful for me." Share enough to let the person know that you are sympathetic, but then go back to listening closely to them.

Giving advice: As a rule of thumb, *only give advice when you are asked*, and always put it in an appropriate, personalized perspective. Unless you are professionally licensed to give advice, keeping it personal allows you to share knowledge without claiming inappropriate authority. For example, "This is what works for me . . ." or "Many people have found this to be helpful…" or "I read an article…you might want to look it up on Internet and check out the information."

Appropriate referrals. Become familiar with professionals in your area who deal with problems your receiver may have. This could include medical and psychological professionals as well as complementary and alternative care practitioners. When giving referrals, offer at least three choices (The Rule of Three) so your receiver can find the practitioner that suits them best.

Basic Hand Positions to Use for Subtle Energy Therapy

Gentle, compassionate touch can be of great assistance to someone who is experiencing discomfort or imbalance. Sometimes, it is all that is needed to help them feel better. Simply holding someone's hand can bring a sense of connection and peace. Yet there are specific touch techniques and placements that can be particularly helpful. The following seven basic hand positions are simple yet powerful. When combined with supportive essential oils, they form a foundation from which to give a helpful subtle energy therapy session.

To use with each hand position, several single essential oils are suggested. Choose the essential oil that is most appropriate at the time. Also included are a visualization and a color exercise for each hand position that will help you keep your intention clear and focused. They are not necessary, but many people find them useful.

The suggested time given to hold each position is only a guideline, and with experience you will know when more or less time is appropriate.

#1 & #2 Open Toes and Close Toes

When you are going to give a subtle energy therapy session to someone, it is a good practice to start with Open Toes, before you begin working with other hand positions. Close Toes is then used at the end of the session. These two hand positions work together to help balance the subtle anatomy and support the process on all levels. If you have used Open Toes, always use Close Toes. Though Open Toes and Close Toes are usually used in 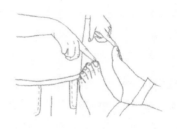 conjunction with other hand positions, they can also be used together on its own.

The tips of the toes correspond to the seven primary energy centers. Because there are five toes and seven energy centers, the connection is not one-to-one. The big toe connects with the First energy center, the baby toe connects with the Sixth and Seventh, and the middle three toes work together on the remaining energy centers (Second, Third, Fourth, and Fifth). The most important consideration is to be aware that touching the tips of each toe, from the biggest down to the smallest, grounds the receiver and gently opens the energy centers to *receive* healing energy. Touching the baby toe up to the big toe also grounds the receiver, and gently closes the energy centers to the degree that is best suited for daily life.

Open Toes and Close Toes are particularly important hand positions because most people have imbalances in their energy centers as they respond to life experiences. Some centers are more opened or closed than others, and there are times when they do not open and close appropriately. Because of trauma, misunderstanding, or confusion, harmful situations may not be recognized, and the energy centers do not respond to protect, as they should. In other cases, healing energy may be unfamiliar, and the energy centers won't open to receive it, or more commonly, only the upper centers will open. In these situations, a combination of intention, energy, and essential oils can be used to open and close each energy center when it is

146

appropriate, creating healthy boundaries and grounded protection for daily living.

Open Toes

The receiver should be lying down on their back, with shoes and socks off.

Using the tips of your index fingers, rest them on the tops of the big toes. Hold for five to ten seconds. Then move your index fingers, simultaneously and sequentially, to the tops of the second, third, fourth, and fifth toes. (Hold each for five to ten seconds.) As you do this, keep the intention of this hand position in your mind, which is to gently open the energy centers in a helpful, harmonious way.

Visualization & Color Exercise: Visualize the opening of each energy center, consecutively, from the First to the Seventh as if they were beautiful flowers. Visualize them in the colors of white, gold, or green.

Close Toes

Place the tips of your index fingers on the tops of the fifth (baby) toes and hold for five to ten seconds. Then touch and hold in succession the fourth, third, and second toes. (Hold each for five to ten seconds.) Lastly, touch the big toes for ten seconds and then hold them, on top and bottom, between your thumbs and index fingers as you send the intention that the energy centers are now closing to a degree that is best for daily living and that the energy received was for the highest good.

Visualization & Color Exercise:
Visualize the energy centers as flowers closing to a bud. Continue to visualize them in white, gold, or green.

Subtle Aromatherapy for Open and Close Toes:
(Each essential oil can be used for both the Open Toes and Close Toes positions.)
1. Chamomile German or Roman deeply relaxes and helps healing energy to be received.
2. Elemi used in Open Toes is grounding and promotes deep relaxation. Used in Close Toes, it helps to bring back everyday reality, even after prolonged or deep relaxation.

3. Lavender balances all the energy centers to the optimum degree of being open or closed.

4. Palmarosa supports all levels of healing and supports the energy centers to receive healing energy.

5. Vetiver grounds and protects all the energy centers.

#3 Forehead Spread

Forehead Spread links the Sixth and Seventh energy centers together and helps to clear the mind so healing energy can be better received. It helps people to integrate new information and insights, so it is useful for those who are in a learning process or cognitive therapy or have a meditation practice. It helps to clear mental confusion, creative blocks, worry, and mental conflict. It is also useful for uncomfortable symptoms in the 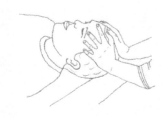 head such as headaches (especially caused by intense study or reading), sinus congestion, eyestrain, neck tension, over thinking, and worry. (Do not use this hand position for migraine headaches.)

The receiver should be lying down, on their back. Place both of your thumbs together, side-by-side, about two inches back from the hairline. Reach your index fingers towards the Sixth (Brow) energy center, as far as is comfortable. Let your other fingers rest into a naturally spaced spread across the forehead, holding gently with symmetrical, even pressure. Hold for one to three minutes, with your intention.

Visualization & Color Exercise:
Visualize sending a calming, deep indigo blue color to the Sixth energy center, and a balancing lavender or white color to the Seventh.

Subtle Aromatherapy for Forehead Spread:
1. Angelica connects to the angelic realm and strengthens spirituality. It grounds the mind and body while opening them to the higher self. It helps to protect the mind during deep relaxation and meditative states.
2. Cedarwood helps to clear and steady the mind and supports the ability to concentrate. It promotes a calm and positive mental state. It helps to strengthen the connection with the Divine.

3. Elemi clears and relaxes the mind, and opens it to grounded, mystical experiences. It helps to balance spiritual and worldly life.

4. Helichrysum helps to clear energy blocks caused by challenging emotions and memories. It activates the right side of the brain (the intuitive and creative mind). It promotes spiritual understanding and the acceptance of difficult experiences.

5. Lavender has a balancing effect on all the energy centers and subtle bodies, and can be energizing or relaxing, depending upon what is needed at the time. It helps to clear energy blocks and brings in positive energy. It promotes mental clarity and awareness and helps to integrate spirituality in everyday life.

6. Rosemary promotes mental clarity and energy and enhances memory and concentration. It helps protect the mind from negative influences. It helps us to remember our spiritual path while inspiring faith. It also helps us to receive and understand spiritual guidance.

7. Rosewood is calming and helps to clear energy blocks. It promotes intuition and gently opens the Seventh (Crown) energy center, as a person is ready.

8. Sandalwood quiets the mind and promotes a deeply receptive, meditative state of mind.

#4 Simple Hold

Simple Hold is designed to work with specific areas of the body, bringing them into balance so that the body's natural healing ability can unfold. The receiver can be in any position that is needed to be comfortable and for you to be able to do the position. The receiver can be sitting, standing, or lying down.

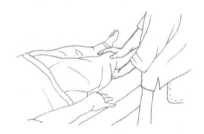

Place your hands on either side of any area on the receiver's body—side-to-side or front to back. It might be an injury, an ache, or a particular energy center. It might be on a leg, arm, joint, finger, toe, or shoulder. Simple Hold can be done with your hands touching the body or off the body in the energy field for situations in which touch would make the body is uncomfortable or for areas that would be inappropriate to touch.

Mentally, hold the intention of healing and visualize a gentle energy wave moving from one of your hands to your other, through the area in need, until the energy flow feels even or continuous, or until you sense that it is finished. If you need to, you can use one hand or one hand on top of the other, to gently send healing energy until you sense the area is full.

As an option to the technique described above, you can hold the area and then every minute or so (or when you sense the need), gently let go of the receiver and shake/flick your hands a few times with the intention of releasing any energy that is ready to be removed from the area. Some practitioners feel this is good for both the person receiving the healing energy and for the person sending it.

NOTE: As you practice, you will discover your way of knowing when the hold is finished. Some people see an image of completion, such as a glass that is full. Others sense a tingling in their hands, and others just "know." There is no right or wrong way to sense this. In the beginning, you may feel more comfortable holding for a prescribed amount of time, and we would recommend three to five minutes.

Visualization & Color Exercise:
Visualize an appropriate color (such as blue or lavender for inflammation, red for increasing circulation, green for balancing, orange for yellow for rejuvenating, or pink for love), moving back and forth between your hands—glowing clear, bright, and strong.

Subtle Aromatherapy for Simple Hold:
When using Simple Hold, essential oils can be chosen four different ways, whichever way feels right to you at the time.

1. Body Parts
Different organs and body parts are associated with and influenced by specific energy centers. (See Chapter 2, as a reference for each energy center, under "Gland association" and "Parts of body influenced.") For example, the thyroid is associated with the Fifth (Throat) energy center. The throat, mouth, ears, neck, and nose are influenced by it.

Identify the body area in need (such as the stomach), identify the energy center associated with it (the Third), and then choose an essential oil that works with the needs of that energy center (such as Rosemary, Orange, or Lavender). To help you choose the oil, we recommend using "The Essential Oils for the Energy Centers" as a reference in Chapter 4. Then use Simple Hold to work with the associated energy center with the intention of benefitting the body part in need.

2. Mental / Emotional Issues

Choose an essential oil that addresses the mental or emotional issue, such as mental fatigue or fear. Other issues might be grief, loneliness, envy, low self-esteem, irritability, sorrow, apathy, confusion, poor memory, or worry. (Chapters 3 and 4 will provide you with the information you need to determine this.) As examples for fear: Orange eases depression and promotes feelings of joy, helping to counteract fear; Cedarwood calms a fearful mind; Ylang Ylang relaxes the body and mind to reduce fear; and Rosemary reduces mental confusion often associated with fear.

Then, work with the energy center that relates to the issue (see Chapter 4 as a reference). As examples, grief is related to the Fourth, low self-esteem is related to the Third, and worry is related to the Sixth. You can also work with the place on the body where the symptoms are felt. Most people feel emotional symptoms in the head, throat, chest, and/or stomach. So, if you are working with someone else, you will need to ask where they feel the emotion. Fear is often felt in the chest, worry in the head, and grief in the head, throat, heart, and stomach areas.

3. Energy Centers

Common imbalances of each energy center are covered in Chapter 4. Choose an essential oil that meets the appropriate need of the energy center. (Chapter 3, which lists the subtle energy properties of fifty-five essential oils, will help you with this. Tea Tree helps to energize when depleted; Black Pepper helps to clear energy blocks; Lavender helps to balance and bring in positive energy; Lemon helps to clear and cleanse; and Pine helps to clear away negative energy strengthen energy flow.) Then, work with the energy center itself, placing your hands on the front and back of the body or by using the one-hand method.

4. Physical Symptoms / Physical Locations

Choose the essential oil that assists with the physical symptom, and then work in the area of the symptom. As examples, use Eucalyptus for respiratory congestion with your hands over the lung area; use Peppermint for indigestion with your hand over the stomach area; and use Rosemary for a tired muscle with your hands over that muscle. (Because these physical level uses of essential oils are not addressed in this book, if you are unfamiliar with the physical uses, we recommend using a reference book that has this information. A few suggestions are *Practical Aromatherapy for Self-care* by Joni Keim and *Aromatherapy: A Lifetime Guide to Healing with Essential Oils* by Valerie Gennari Cooksley.

Simple Hold Positions to Help Specific Situations

1. Hands cupped over the eyes: Relieves anxiety, reduces stress, relaxes, and promotes mental clarity.
2. Hands covering the temples: Relieves worry, reduces stress, and promotes calmness and mental clarity.
3. Hands covering the back of the head: Reduces fear and worry, relieves stress, and promotes a sense of well-being.
4. Hands over the throat: Relieves anger, resentment, and frustration, and promotes feelings of security.
5. Hands over the heart: Promotes relaxation, comforts, and reduces stress.
6. Hands over the liver/stomach: Reduces stress and anxiety, relieves frustration, and promotes self-confidence.
7. Hands over the lower stomach: Releases anger and fear and promotes creativity.
8. Hands cupping over the ears: Promotes receptivity to inner and outer guidance.
9. Hands on the ankles: Releases tension and stress.
10. Hands on the knees: Releases tension and stress, releases unpleasant emotions, and promotes forgiveness.
11. Hands on the wrists: Releases tension and stress, and promotes creative expression.
12. Hands on elbows: Releases tension and stress, and promotes interaction with one's environment.
13. Hands on the shoulders: Releases tension and stress, and helps to motivate.

#5 Filling

This is a gently energizing technique that helps to increase/restore physical, mental, or emotional vitality. It helps to relieve fatigue, emotional exhaustion, symptoms of burn-out, and stress.

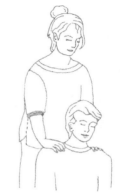

The receiver can be sitting in a chair or lying down, whichever is more comfortable for them. This technique is well suited for more public places when reclining is not possible or appropriate.

Place your palms on the shoulders or feet of the receiver. Visualize the earth's energy being drawn in through the bottom of your feet and filling your Fourth (Heart) energy center. Imagine it moving to your Fifth (Throat) energy center, down your arms, and then out your hands to fill the receiver. Hold for five minutes, with your intention for their health and well-being.

Visualization & Color Exercise:
Visualize a soft red, medium orange, or sun yellow, flowing out of your hands and filling the receiver's body from feet up or shoulders down until their entire body is full. Then visualize it overflowing out of the top of their head, or out the bottoms of their feet, filling the subtle bodies.

Subtle Aromatherapy for Filling:
1. Lavender balances and can be gently energizing when needed.
2. Orange fills with uplifting joy.
3. Pine increases energy in the subtle bodies.
4. Mandarin uplifts and promotes youthful joy.
5. Rosemary relieves mental fatigue and energizes.

#6 & 7 Combing and Smoothing the Energy Field

Combing and Smoothing are used together and are typically the last step in a session. They are designed to promote a general sense of well-being by soothing, comforting, sealing, and protecting the subtle bodies. They help to replenish the energy field's boundaries, and remove debris that has been released during the subtle energy therapy session.

Combing. The receiver should be lying down on their back. Hold your hands three to twelve inches away from the receiver's body, directing your fingertips towards their body. Your fingers should have space between them, as if they were teeth in a comb. Imagine white light coming from each of your fingertips, as they comb through and straighten out any tangles in the energy field. Begin at the 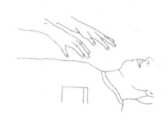 head and move down one side of the body and then the other, using long, steady strokes. At the feet, comb out and beyond the body, and then shake your hands to shake off and release any energy debris that has been collected.

Visualization & Color Exercise:
While combing, visualize streams of white, pink, or gold light coming from each finger as the fingers comb through the energy field.

Smoothing. Hold your hands about twelve inches away from the receiver's body. Slightly cup your hands with your fingers close together. Begin at the head and move down one side of the body and then the other, using long, smoothing strokes. At the feet, smooth out and beyond the body. Remember to periodically shake or flick your hands towards the ground to release any energy debris that has been collected.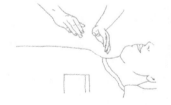

Visualization & Color Exercise:
While smoothing, imagine your cupped palms filled with white, pink, or gold light. If you prefer, you can use a color that coordinates with the essential oil used such as rose for Rose oil, lavender for Lavender oil, yellow-orange for Palmarosa, or a burnished golden brown for Vetiver.

Subtle Aromatherapy for Combing and Smoothing the Energy Field:
1. Rose gently fills holes in the energy field. It also grounds the energy centers.
2. Lavender smoothes and balances the energy centers and the energy field.
3. Palmarosa has a gentle nature that supports the healing process.
4. Vetiver grounds and stabilizes.

Giving a Subtle Energy Therapy Session

It is appropriate to offer a subtle energy therapy session whenever someone would like one and you have the time, energy, and are in state of mind to give one. People receive sessions for all sorts of reasons—physical symptoms, emotional upset, a desire for deep relaxation, a need for energizing, or the comfort of safe, compassionate touch. We believe the intelligence of the receiver's physical body and subtle anatomy guides the energy coming through your hands to be of the quality that is needed and will be of the most benefit.

Preparing to Give a Subtle Energy Therapy Session

Whether you have a special place in which you can give subtle energy therapy sessions or you use whatever space is available, always take a few moments to dedicate the area by *setting sacred space*: clear and cleanse, bring in positive energy, establish boundaries, and ask for guidance, as described in Chapter 4.

After you have done the exercises, "Center in Your Breath" and "Prepare Your Hands" (Chapter 2), you are ready to begin.
1. First, relax your body, your facial muscles, and especially the muscles around your eyes. Soften your visual focus so that it becomes diffused and expanded to include peripheral vision. This helps create a more intuitive and receptive state of mind.
2. Put a drop of a grounding essential oil on your feet, such as Frankincense or Patchouli. Then put a drop of Lavender on your hands to help open them to healing energy.
3. Say a simple prayer/intention to attract the most beneficial energy, out loud or silently. A favorite is, "May this person and I be healed and filled with light." Always be clear about your intention for the session, as discussed in Chapter 2.

4. Invite the receiver into the dedicated area, and if you haven't already discussed what it is they want, take a few minutes to do that now, using your active listening skills. This helps you and your receiver focus on what is needed at this time.

5. Ask the receiver to lie down on their back. A massage table is ideal but a bed, table, or the floor, will also work. Whatever it is, be sure that both of you are comfortable. Some people like a pillow under both their neck and knees for support. Cover your receiver with a sheet, and a blanket, if necessary. Encourage them to let you know if they become too hot or too cold so you can remove or add blankets. Healing energy often changes the temperature of the body. NOTE: If lying down is not physically possible for the receiver, the hand positions can be done with the receiver sitting in a comfortable chair.

You are now ready to give a subtle energy therapy session. Be considerate in your approach to your receiver. Because the subtle bodies extend several inches to several feet beyond their physical body, contact is made as soon as your body and the receiver's bodies are close to each other—*before* actual physical contact. Abrupt or harsh approaches are jarring and can be unpleasant. Be calm and gentle. When you are finished with the session, slowly and gently disconnect, and leave their energy field the same way, slowly and gently, with respect.

The following are descriptions of ten different subtle energy sessions designed for different purposes. For children, seniors, or someone who is ill, decrease the recommended time by half. In each type of session, preparing for and ending the session are the same. See Appendix III for suggestions for more subtle energy therapy sessions. The essential oils used in the following sessions are applied as anointing oils, unless otherwise mentioned. See Chapter 4 for recipes.

A Session for Relaxation and Stress Relief

1. *Open Toes.* One to two minutes. Put Lavender and/or Chamomile Roman anointing oil on your hands to help your receiver relax and be receptive to the session.

2. *Forehead Spread.* Three minutes. Put a drop of Frankincense anointing oil on the top of the receiver's head to calm and comfort. Rest your fingers in place on their forehead. Imagine and visualize a relaxing blue color light is moving out from your fingers and palms, filling their body and then moving out of their body via their fingers and toes.

3. *Simple Hold.* Two to four minutes. Add a drop of a grounding anointing oil to your hands such as Frankincense or Cedarwood. Gently hold the ankles and send healing energy for one to two minutes. Then move your hands to the bottoms of the feet and send energy for another one to two minutes. Imagine and visualize their physical body deeply relaxed, all the energy centers balanced and in harmony, and that the subtle bodies are gently glowing with peace and harmony.

4. *Close Toes.* Two minutes. Touch each toe, beginning with the smallest and moving up to the big toes. Visualize the energy centers closing to the size that will be best for your receiver during the rest of their day.

5. *Combing and Smoothing.* Two minutes. Mist your receiver with Lavender or Rose, and gently comb and smooth their energy field.

A Session for Energizing

1. *Open Toes.* One to two minutes. Put Lavender anointing oil on your hands to help your receiver be receptive to the session.

2. *Filling.* Three minutes. Put Pine anointing oil on your hands to increase energy in the physical and subtle bodies and to rejuvenate. Then place your hands on your receiver's shoulders. Imagine and visualize their body and energy field glowing with an energizing light— red, orange, or yellow.

3. *Close Toes.* Two minutes. Touch each toe, beginning with the smallest and moving up to the big toes. Visualize the energy centers closing to the size that will be best for your receiver during the rest of their day.

4. *Combing and Smoothing.* Two minutes. Mist your receiver with Lavender or Rose, and gently comb and smooth their energy field.

A Session for Relieving Aches

1. *Open Toes.* One to two minutes. Put Lavender or Chamomile Roman anointing oil on your hands to help your receiver relax and be receptive to the session.

2. The hand position you use depends on whether it is a headache or an ache somewhere else on the body.

For a headache: *Forehead Spread.* Three minutes. Put a drop of Lavender or Chamomile German anointing oil on the top of the receiver's head to calm and support healing. Rest your fingers very gently and lightly in place on their forehead. Imagine and visualize a soothing blue color light moving out from your fingers and palms, and filling their Sixth energy center, head, and neck. (Do not use this technique on a migraine headache.)

OR

For an ache on the body: *Simple Hold*. Two positions—two minutes each.

First, hold the energy center or centers that the ache is associated with. (This information is available in Chapter 2.) As examples, a throat issue is associated with the Fifth energy center, a stomach issue is associated with the Third energy center, and a lower back issue is associated with the Second and Third energy centers. (If there is more than one center that you are working with, begin with the lower one first.) Imagine and visualize the color associated with the energy center flowing from your hands to fill the center.

Second, move your hands to the area that is experiencing the ache. If it is not tender, you can touch the area. If it is tender, hold your hands about six inches above it. Imagine and visualize a soothing blue color light flowing from your hands and filling the area. Gradually visualize the color changing to a warm rose and then a soft lavender.

3. *Close Toes*. Two minutes. Touch each toe, beginning with the smallest and moving up to the big toes. Visualize the energy centers closing to the size that will be best for your receiver during the rest of their day.

4. *Combing and Smoothing*. Two minutes. Mist your receiver with Lavender or Rose, and gently comb and smooth their energy field.

A Session to Feel Safe and Secure

1. *Open Toes*. One to two minutes. Put Lavender and/or Chamomile Roman anointing oil on your hands to help your receiver relax and be receptive to the session.

2. *Forehead Spread*. Three minutes. Put a drop of Sandalwood anointing oil on the top of the receiver's head to calm and comfort. Rest your fingers in place on their forehead. Imagine and visualize a clear red color light moving out from your fingers and palms, slowly moving through their body, and then moving out of their body via their fingers and toes.

3. *Simple Hold*. Two minutes. Put a drop of Frankincense anointing oil on the palm of each of your hands to promote a sense of security. Hold your hands off the body six to twelve inches over their First (Root) energy center. Visualize a clear red color light being sent into the center, and imagine it filling with that light and becoming balanced and strong.

4. *Filling*. Two minutes. Put a drop of Sandalwood anointing oil on the palms of each of your hands for comfort and strength. Then place your

hands on your receiver's feet or shoulders. Visualize a golden color light flowing from your hands to fill their entire body.

5. *Simple Hold.* Two minutes. Return to the feet. Put one hand on each foot. Imagine a rich, dark green color flowing from your hands to fill their whole body with grounding, earth energy.

6. *Close Toes.* Two minutes. Touch each toe, beginning with the smallest and moving up to the big toes. Visualize the energy centers closing to the size that will be best for your receiver during the rest of their day.

7. *Combing and Smoothing.* Two minutes. Mist your receiver with Lavender or Rose, and gently comb and smooth their energy field.

A Session to Enhance Creativity

1. *Open Toes.* One to two minutes. Put Lavender and/or Chamomile Roman anointing oil on your hands to help your receiver relax and be receptive to the session.

2. *Forehead Spread.* Two minutes. Put a drop of Jasmine anointing oil on the top of the receiver's head and on the palms of your hands to promote creativity and heighten the senses. Rest your fingers in place on their forehead. Imagine and visualize an inspiring orange color light moving out from your fingers and palms, through their body, and out their fingers and toes.

3. *Simple Hold.* Four positions, one and a half minutes for each position. First, place your hands over the receiver's Second (Sacral) energy center. Visualize this center filled with a clear orange color light and generating creativity and ingenuity.

Second, move your hands over their Third (Solar Plexus) energy center and hold them there to strengthen confidence, while visualizing a golden sun.

Third, put a drop of Bergamot anointing oil on the palms of both your hands. Move your hands to their Fourth (Heart) energy center, and visualize a pink, rose, or green flower opening. Imagine any energy block gently clearing away beneath your hands.

Fourth, with Chamomile German anointing oil on your palms, put your hands over their Fifth (Throat) energy center. Visualize a beautiful blue flower opening and imagine this energy center generating creativity and expression.

4. *Close Toes.* Two minutes. Touch each toe, beginning with the smallest and moving up to the big toes. Visualize the energy centers closing to the size that will be best for your receiver during the rest of their day.

5. *Combing and Smoothing*. Two minutes. Mist your receiver with Lavender or Rose, and gently comb and smooth their energy field.

A Session for Confidence and Self-Esteem

1. *Open Toes*. One to two minutes. Put Lavender and/or Chamomile Roman anointing oil on your hands to help your receiver relax and be receptive to the session.

2. *Forehead Spread*. Two minutes. Put a drop of Lemon anointing oil on the top of the receiver's head uplift and strengthen self esteem. Rest your fingers in place on their forehead. Imagine and visualize a clear yellow color light flowing from your fingers and palms, through their body, and out their fingers and toes.

3. *Simple Hold*. Two minutes. Put a drop of Petitgrain anointing oil on your hands and place them over their Third energy center to promote self-esteem, confidence, and optimism. Imagine this area filling with a clear, golden color—like the sun in its warmth and light.

4. *Close Toes*. Two minutes. Touch each toe, beginning with the smallest and moving up to the big toes. Visualize the energy centers closing to the size that will be best for your receiver during the rest of their day.

5. *Combing and Smoothing*. Two minutes. Mist your receiver with Lavender or Rose, and gently comb and smooth their energy field.

A Session for a Joyful Heart

1. *Open Toes*. One to two minutes. Put Lavender anointing oil on your hands to help your receiver relax and be receptive to the session.

2. *Simple Hold*. Two minutes. Place a drop of Ylang Ylang anointing oil on the palm of one of your hands and place it over their Second (Sacral) energy center to release any fear that may be impeding joyfulness. Place a drop of Rose anointing oil on your other hand and place it over their Fourth (Heart) energy center to support it on all levels—physical, emotional, mental, and spiritual. Imagine and visualize these centers as healthy, strong and clear, and stay there until you feel a sense that they are both connected and balanced with each other.

3. *Simple Hold*. Two minutes. Put Orange anointing oil on both your hands and hold them over the Fourth (Heart) energy center to uplift and promote joy. Imagine and visualize a beautiful, joyful heart that is uplifted, positive, and at peace.

4. *Close Toes*. Two minutes. Touch each toe, beginning with the smallest and moving up to the big toes. Visualize the energy centers closing to the size that will be best for your receiver during the rest of their day.

5. *Combing and Smoothing.* Two minutes. Mist your receiver with Lavender or Rose, and gently comb and smooth their energy field.

A Session for Positive Communication

1. *Open Toes.* One to two minutes. Put Lavender and/or Chamomile Roman anointing oil on your hands to help your receiver relax and be receptive to the session.

2. *Forehead Spread.* Two minutes. Put a drop of Orange anointing oil on the top of the receiver's head and on the palms of your hands. Rest your fingers in place on their forehead. Imagine and visualize a sky-blue color light flowing from your fingers and palms, through their body, and out their fingers and toes.

3. *Simple Hold.* Two minutes. Place one of your hands over their Second (Sacral) energy center to support a deepening trust in life and relationships. On your other hand, place a drop of Chamomile German anointing oil and rest it on their Fifth (Throat) energy center to promote healthy, positive communication. Send balancing energy into each center visualizing an orange color light into the Second energy center and sky-blue color light into the Fifth energy center. Hold this position until you sense that the two centers are connected and balanced with each other. This hold will assist the receiver in understanding what they want/need (Second energy center) so that they can positively and truthfully communicate it (Fifth energy center).

4. *Close Toes.* Two minutes. Touch each toe, beginning with the smallest and moving up to the big toes. Visualize the energy centers closing to the size that will be best for your receiver during the rest of their day.

5. *Combing and Smoothing.* Two minutes. Mist your receiver with Lavender or Rose, and gently comb and smooth their energy field.

A Session for Mental Clarity and Energy

1. *Open Toes.* One to two minutes. Put Lavender anointing oil on your hands to help your receiver be receptive to the session.

2. *Forehead Spread.* Four minutes. Put a drop of Rosemary anointing oil on the top of the receiver's head and on the palms of your hands to clear and energize the mind. Rest your fingers in place on their forehead. Imagine and visualize that a clear indigo color light is moving out from your fingers and palms, through their body, and out their fingers and toes. Then imagine and visualize the receiver's Sixth (Brow) energy center to be healthy and balanced, glowing with an indigo color

light. Imagine and visualize your receiver's mind to be clear and energized.

3. *Close Toes*. Two minutes. Touch each toe, beginning with the smallest and moving up to the big toes. Visualize the energy centers closing to the size that will be best for your receiver during the rest of their day.

4. *Combing and Smoothing*. Two minutes. Mist your receiver with Lavender or Rose, and gently comb and smooth their energy field.

A Session for Spiritual Rejuvenation

1. *Open Toes*. One to two minutes. Put Lavender and/or Chamomile Roman anointing oil on your hands to help your receiver relax and be receptive to the session.

2. *Forehead Spread*. Three minutes. To support this spiritual rejuvenation at an appropriate level, place a drop of Rosewood anointing oil on the top of the receiver's head and on the palms of your hands. Imagine their Seventh energy center slowly opening at an appropriate pace, like a great, violet color flower.

3. *Simple Hold*. Two minutes. Put a drop of Sandalwood anointing oil on both your hands and hold them over their Seventh energy center to support spiritual development. Imagine and visualize filling this center with a clear lavender color light that supports spiritual renewal and transformation.

4. *Close Toes*. Two minutes. Touch each toe, beginning with the smallest and moving up to the big toes. Visualize the energy centers closing to the size that will be best for your receiver during the rest of their day.

5. *Combing and Smoothing*. Two minutes. Mist your receiver with Lavender or Rose, and gently comb and smooth their energy field.

Ending A Subtle Energy Therapy Session

When you are finished with a subtle energy therapy session, quietly let your receiver know that you are going to go wash your hands, and they may just lay comfortably until you come back. Leave softly and gently. As you wash your hands, imagine that any energy that you might have picked up from the receiver is running down the drain with the soap and water.

Re-enter the room quietly and respectfully and assist your receiver in sitting up. Offer a glass of cool water to drink. This has a grounding effect and helps them to orient to their surroundings. Suggest they drink plenty of water during the day to assist in the integration of the effects of the session. These effects will continue over the next few days. Before they get up, make sure they are well grounded. If a bit unsteady, have them take a sniff of Rosemary or Lemon, and put a drop of Cedarwood or Frankincense anointing oil on the bottom of their feet. It is your responsibility to be certain they are well grounded and re-oriented before they leave.

Ask them to tell you briefly how they are doing. A brief conversation at this time can help them ground in ordinary consciousness. However, a lengthy discussion would not be desirable as it could dissipate the energy. If they have questions or comments that require more attention, let them know that you can talk to them in the following day or two.

After the receiver has left, take the time to adjust *yourself* back to ordinary reality. Clear and cleanse the area again and imagine that *you* are cleared and cleansed as well. Return the room or area to its normal state. Offer a prayer of gratitude for all the gifts just given and received. As you have given, you have also received beyond measure.

After a Subtle Energy Therapy Session

To further support the unfolding and deepening of a subtle energy therapy session, it is helpful to give your receiver an anointing oil to take home. Every time they smell or apply it, it will support the beneficial changes that have occurred during the session, and the aroma will direct the receiver's memory to the experience and intention of healing. In this way, the essential oils are working as psychological support as well as a vibrational medicine tool.

When at home, the receiver can repeat some of the techniques used during their session to assist their energy centers. They can smell the anointing oil from the bottle or place it on a tissue to inhale when needed or desired. They can put a drop on their hands and hold it over an energy center with the intent to balance or place a drop on their body at the location of the energy center or body area in need of help.

You may also suggest visualization techniques that can help your receiver work on their energy centers at home. As they apply the anointing oil, instruct them to:
1. Visualize the energy center's associated color flowing from their anointing oil into the center, creating balance and harmony. For example, visualize a beautiful, sky blue color flowing from Chamomile German anointing oil into the Fifth (Throat) energy center.

2. Visualize the energy center gleaming with its clear color, round, open, moving clockwise, and being healthy and balanced.

3. Encourage them to create a meaningful image to represent the energy center as being strong, healthy, and balanced. It may be an animal, a plant, a nature scene, or a personally meaningful symbol. Visualize the image being securely planted in that energy center, bringing wellness. As examples: Mother Earth in the First (Root) energy center; an opened, orange flower in the Second (Sacral) energy center; a brilliant yellow sun in the Third (Solar Plexus) energy center; a peaceful, green meadow with pink flowers in bloom for the Fourth (Heart) energy center; an expansive, blue sky in the Fifth (Throat) energy center; a dream appearing in rich, indigo blue in the Sixth (Brow) energy center; an angel surrounded by a violet light in the Seventh (Crown) energy center; a soft pink rose for the Hands centers; and a large, strong dark green tree firmly planted in the ground for the Feet centers.

Case Studies with Ruah Bull, Ph.D.

Ruah Bull, co-author of this book, has worked for twenty-five years in the healing arts as a hypnotherapist, energy healer, and spiritual director. The following are interesting case studies and examples of what can be done with subtle energy therapy, intention, and essential oils.

1) "A man had severe arthritis in his left shoulder, wrist, and hand. I was using Simple Hold to help him send more energy through his arm, but the energy was not moving. I put a clearing mist of Cedarwood, Eucalyptus, and Juniper on my hands, and asked him to smell it. He said he loved the aroma and felt it went deeply into his body. The energy then began to move, and the client reported a soothing warmth running down his arm. After giving him a blend to use at home and helping him develop an image to affirm the sensation, he now comes in monthly rather than weekly, and reports with delight that for the first time in years, he has greater movement in his fingers."

2) "An elderly woman living in a nursing home was feeling depressed and apathetic. She reported that she was physically exhausted and didn't want to get up out of her easy chair or leave her room. I put

Orange anointing oil on my hands, placed my hands on her knees as I sat facing her in her chair, and used the Filling technique as we chatted. After about fifteen minutes, she reported feeling a bit more energy, and was willing to go to the dining room for her meal. After experimenting with various essential oils, we discovered that she particularly loved Lavender, both for its aroma and the pleasant memories it brought back to her. The nursing home staff agreed to spray Lavender in her room several times a day, and they reported that her mood greatly improved. They also noted that she seemed to be sleeping more comfortably at night, and they wanted to try aromatherapy with other residents."

3) "A deeply spiritual woman was distressed by her need to fire an employee. She was afraid to hurt the person's feelings, but also believed that she had to be truthful about why the person was being released. Just before her meeting with the employee, we made a blend of both Chamomile German and Roman for gentle, truthful communication, with a drop of Bergamot to activate the Heart energy center, and a bit of Frankincense to ground. We used it with the Filling technique on her Fourth and Fifth energy centers. Afterward, she felt better able to hold her ground and speak her truth in both a clear, respectful, and compassionate manner. She reported later that although it had still been difficult for her, she had been able to act from her spiritual beliefs and treat both herself and the other person with dignity and respect. The following week when we met, she was remembering other difficult situations when she had been attacked for speaking the truth. We blended Rosemary, Fennel, and Juniper to make an anointing oil. I placed it on my hands and her Third (Solar Plexus) energy center and did a Simple Hold on that center for about ten minutes. She was able to release many old feelings that she had taken on from other people— especially their anger—and she reported feeling much lighter than she had in a long time."

4) "A woman with pre-menstrual syndrome (PMS) had not been able to find much relief. In a session, we blended Rose and Jasmine, and worked on her Second (Sacral) energy center with Simple Hold. She began to weep after getting in touch with all the messages she had received as a little girl about menstruation being a "curse," and how that had translated into dislike of her female body. She was able to take these issues to her therapist, and by integrating energy work and

aromatherapy with her therapy, she was able to experience both a deep psychological healing as well as much relief from her PMS symptoms. On her Second (Sacral) energy center we used Rose and Jasmine to support the feminine. On her Fourth (Heart) energy center we used Rose and Bergamot to promote self-love and love of her body."

An Exercise with a Hand Position and an Essential Oil

1. Pick one of the subtle energy hand positions, practice it on a receiver, and notice what happens. What does the receiver experience? What do you experience?

2. Now place an appropriate essential oil on your hands and practice the same hand position. What does the receiver notice? What is different from the first exercise? What is the same? What do you notice the second time?

3. Experiment with the different techniques and essential oils and discover how they complement each other.

NOTE: It can be helpful to teach your receiver about what it means to notice the effects of a particular oil or technique. Let them know that there may be a change in feelings—a different temperature (hot or cold), or a different sensation (tight, loose, relaxed, hard, blocked, flowing, empty, tingling, heavy, or light). They may perceive a color, texture, or see an image. Some people hear things. Others will not perceive anything at all. Whatever happens for them is right for them at that time. Be supportive, no matter what they experience.

Afterword

You now have all the information you need to begin using and experiencing the transformative, healing art of subtle aromatherapy and subtle energy therapy. We hope that your practice of this work will bring you the same possibilities for joy, healing, and spiritual growth that it has given to us. We wish you peace and wisdom.

"People won't remember what you've said, and people won't remember what you've done but people will remember how you made them feel."

--Author unknown

Appendix I:
The Subtle Properties of Uncommon Essential Oils

The following essential oils are uncommon and often unknown. In this revised and updated edition of *Aromatherapy and Subtle Energy Techniques*, we did not include them with those that are commonly used (Chapter 3) because they can be difficult to find and many of them have unusual and sometimes unpleasant aromas. However, we did not want to exclude them, as they are unique and special, and there is little information about their subtle energy properties elsewhere. Each one resonates in a specific way with one or more of the energy centers, as explained in their descriptions below.

If you want to use one of these essential oils but the aroma is unpleasant to you, try using a very tiny amount on a tissue and inhale the aroma from a distance and/or very briefly. You can also try blending it with a more pleasant-smelling essential oil, such as Lavender. Be aware, however, that if you combine it with another essential oil, you will also be combining the subtle energy properties, so be sure they are compatible and have the properties you want. (Lavender is often a perfect choice, as it tends to amplify the qualities of other essential oils you are using.)

Ammi Visnaga (*Ammi visnaga*)
Sixth: Supports the development of intuition by increasing the energy in the left-brain. Increases the ability to creatively visualize. Integrates left-brain reality with right-brain imagination. Brings clarity and objectivity to intuitive information.

Amyris (*Amyris balsamifera*)
Sixth: Supports the development of the right-brain to increase creativity and imagination.

Artemisia (*Artemisia afra*)
First and Second: Helps us to fully connect and embrace the earthly experience. Good for people who think that being spiritual means rejecting the world.

Azalea (*Azalea*)
General: Helps to release emotional energy blocks and promote emotional wisdom.
Seventh: Releases emotions lodged in the astral body that interferes with receiving spiritual guidance. Helps us to identify our spiritual path.

Birch (*Betula alba*)
General: Clears and cleanses. Protects and releases fear.
Third: Promotes courage and integrity.
Sixth: Promotes focus and concentration.

Broom (*Spartium junceum*)
First: Helps to ground people that are too much "in their heads."
Seventh: Brings spiritual sustenance to people that are over-attached to the material world.

Bucco Leaves (*Barosma buchulina*)
First: Promotes a sense of stability and being well-grounded in most circumstances, including those that are uncomfortable or unfamiliar.

Cabreuva (*Myrocarpus fastigiatus*)
General: Brings all of the energy centers into balance and harmony with each other. Clears and cleanses. Seals and protects the energy field to promote healthy boundaries.

Cajeput (*Melaleuca cajeputi*)
General: Develops child-like devotion and trust in the universe.

Calamus (*Acorus calamus*)
General: Good for any kind of spiritual/intuitive work. Brings information directly from the Seventh energy center so that it can be clearly understood by the mind (Sixth energy center) and communicated effectively (Fifth energy center).

Carvi (*Carum carvi*)
Fifth: Assists with all issues related to this energy center. Promotes clear communication and good listening. Facilitates 'hearing' body/mind/spirit wisdom.

Cascarilla (*Croton niveous*)
Third: Supports personal will and promotes integrity and self-esteem.

Cedrella (*Cedrella odorata*)
Third: Acts as a general tonic. Clears and cleanses to release negativity while promoting self-esteem, will power, and integrity.

Champaca (*Michelia champaca*)
General: Balances and rejuvenates the energy field and energy centers.
Third, Fourth, Fifth, Sixth, and Seventh: Assists these energy centers, as a group, to move to a higher level of spiritual development.
Sixth: Opens the mind to Divine energy and information. Supports development of intuition.

Cistus (*Cistus ladaniferus*)
Fifth: Promotes ability to "hear" spiritual messages.
Sixth: Promotes intuitive visions and dreams.
Seventh: Assists in receiving clear spiritual guidance.

Costus Root (*Saussurea lappa*)
General: Balances all the energy centers. Balances and cleanses the etheric body to provide the healthiest possible blueprint for the physical body. Good for grounding after meditation.

Croton Anisatum (*Croton anisatum*)
General: Balances and helps to ease challenging emotions, such as fear, anger, and greed so that actions can be taken from a calm, centered awareness. Activates the "spiritual warrior."

Copaiva Balm (*Copaifera reticulata*)
Sixth and Seventh: Links these two energy centers, to align the human mind with the spirituality. Supports mindful, higher consciousness.

Curry Leaves (*Murraya koenigii*)
Seventh: Promotes spiritual development. Helps to open us to Divine guidance.

Cypriol (*Cyperus scariosus*)
General: Helps find a positive perspective in difficult times and situations.
Sixth: Helps to see clearly when experiencing difficult emotions.

Elecampane (*Inula helenium*)
General: Clears, cleanses, and protects the astral body.
Second: Assists in balancing all the issues related to this energy center—creativity, emotions, and sexuality.

Erigeron (*Conyza canadensis*)
General: Helps in discovering one's life purpose.
Sixth and Seventh: Gently opens these energy centers to allow spiritual energy to come in.

Eriocephalus (*Eriocephalus africanus*)
General: Balances and grounds. Helps to integrate meditative experiences. Helps us to slow down mentally and physically so we can be more spiritually attuned.

Fokienia (*Fokienia hodginsii*)
General: Balances and grounds all the energy centers to promote the development of courage, integrity, focus, purpose, and compassion. Especially useful during times of stress.

Frangipani (*Plumeria rubia*)
General: Promotes healing in our relationship with the feminine, especially the mother. Helps us embrace the earthly life.
First: Helps to heal our relationship with Mother Earth and embrace the earthly life. Helps to connect our earthly life with Spirit.
Fourth: Helps expand our capacity to nurture others.
Seventh: Promotes an awareness of the feminine aspect of the Divine. Helps us to spiritually embrace earthly life.

Galbanum (*Ferula galbaniflua*)
First: Promotes a sense of stability.
Third: Promotes fortitude and personal direction.
Sixth: Promotes ability to concentrate. Calms and balances the mind.
Seventh: Promotes trust and faith in Spirit.

Galgant Root (*Alpinia galanga*)
Third: Helps personal will to become balanced and healthy. Promotes personal integrity.

Gingerlily (*Hedychium spicatum*)
Fourth: Strengthens the Heart energy center to be able to experience more love. Promotes compassion.

Golden Rod (*Solidago canadensis*)
Fifth: Helps to balance this energy center to improve the ability to communicate well—both listening and speaking.
Sixth and Seventh: Promotes receptivity to spiritual guidance.

Greenland Moss (*Ledum groenlandicum*)
Sixth: Helps to strengthen memory and promote clarity of thought. Integrates left-brain rationality with right-brain intuition to enhance productivity and creativity.
Seventh: Promotes balanced spirituality.

Guaiac Wood (*Bulnesia sarmienti*)
General: Balances all the energy centers. Integrates spirituality and personal will.
Third and Seventh: Encourages spirituality to influence personal will. Helps to prepare the personality for spiritual development.
Second and Fourth: Helps develop the capacity for healthy surrender.

Gurjum (*Dipteropcarpus turbinatua*)
Sixth and Seventh: Supports meditative states. Activates the intuitive mind. Helps to open these energy centers to receive and integrate spiritual energy.

Hay (*Hierochela alpina*)
Sixth and Seventh: Supports meditation. Promotes connecting with intuitive and spiritual guidance, especially from the plant kingdom.

Hyssop (*Hyssopus officinalis decumbens*)
General: Clears negative energy and protects.
Second: Provides protection from others' moods and emotions. Eases feelings of guilt. Promotes healthy emotional boundaries.

Fourth: Promotes acceptance and eases feelings of grief. Allows for the development of detached compassion.
Sixth: Supports ability to discern.
Seventh: Enhances spirituality.

Kanuka (*Leptospermum ericoides*)
General: Balances all the energy centers. Increases feelings of joy and an abundant life.

Lantana (*Lantana camara*)
Fifth: Promotes the ability to hear spiritual guidance (clairaudience) with discernment. Helps to develop ability to hear one's inner voice.

Larch (*Larix laricina*)
General: Promotes clarity of thought and feelings. Energizes and uplifts.

Leptospermum (*Leptospermum citratum*)
Sixth: Assists the modern person to understand and integrate the ancient wisdom of indigenous people.

Lovage (*Levisticum officinale*)
First: Grounds and centers. Opens the First (Root) and Feet energy centers to receive and integrate earth energy.
Hands: Opens Hands energy centers so that healing earth energy can be sent without draining the one's energy.

Magnolia (*Magnolia grandiflora*)
Fourth: Increases the ability to give and receive love.
Fifth: Increases the ability to speak and hear about love.
Sixth and Seventh: Teaches the love and wisdom of Spirit.

Mangoginger (*Cureuma amada*)
Second: Promotes playful sensuality and sexual joy. Reduces fear and other effects of emotional and physical traumas pertaining to sexuality.

Mastic (*Pistacia lentiscus*)
Seventh: Supports a direct and close connection with Divine guidance and capacity to integrate that guidance.

Mimosa (*Acacia dealbata*)
Fourth: Gently opens the Heart energy center to receive love.
Sixth: Promotes gentle, intuitive dreams. Enhances intuition.

Monarda (*Monarda didyma*)
Seventh: A spiritual gatekeeper that allows us to perceive, receive, and/or understand information for which we are ready. Prevents spiritual confusion and overwhelm.

Myrtle (*Myrtus communis*)
General: Provides protection during major life transitions.
7th: Promotes a connection with Spirit, especially during times of transition.
Fourth: Promotes acceptance. Protects.

Narcissus (*Narcissus poeticus*)
Second: Promotes creativity.
Third: Promotes self-awareness.
Fourth: Helps to ease grief and hopelessness. Helps to heal emotional wounds. Promotes empathy and self-forgiveness.
Sixth: Inspires. Promotes intuitive visions.

Niaouli (*Melaleuca quinquenervia*)
General: Powerful protection against negative outside influences.

Nigella Seeds (*Nigella sativa*)
General: Grounds, balances, and protects all the energy centers.

Opopanax (*Commiphora erythraea*)
General: Helps to heal physical, emotional, mental, and spiritual wounds. Provides physical and psychological protection.
Sixth: Promotes wisdom and understanding.
Seventh: Helps prepare us for receiving mystical wisdom.

Pastinak (*Pastinaca sativa*)
Sixth: Supports the left-brain, bringing in the best qualities of "common sense"—clear, calm, grounded, practical, and logical.

Pistache (*Pistacia lentiscus*)
General: Strengthens our physical energy so that the body can tolerate and integrate greater spiritual energy.

Santolina (*Santolina chamaecyparissus*)
General: Supports feminine nature. Helps to access the innocent joy of a young woman and the experienced wisdom of maturity.

Savory, Winter (*Satureja montana*)
General: Helps us to appreciate, connect, and understand the wisdom and spirituality found in nature.
Second and Seventh: Links these two energy centers, providing spiritual wisdom through the emotional realm.

Sea Fennel (*Cribimum maritimum*)
General: Helps to give us strength and focus to deal with challenging situations.
Third: Acts as a "cloak of power." Promotes a sense of being protected and having appropriate personal power. Promotes healthy, personal boundaries.

Spikenard (*Nardostachys jatamansi*)
General: Promotes a sense of heart-centered wholeness.
Third: Promotes courage and resolution.
Fourth: Comforts and balances the emotions of the heart, especially for people who take on the cares of the world. Promotes compassion and the forgiveness of self and others. Helps to develop detached compassion.
Fifth: Promotes compassionate communication. Helps communication between humans and animals.
Seventh: Promotes love and devotion for the Divine.

St. John's Wort (*Hypericum perforatum*)
Sixth: Helps to open the mind to receive intuitive dreams. Helps us to understand the personal meaning of our dreams.

Tolu-Balsam (*Myroxylon balsamum*)
General: Helps us to feel that life is precious and sweet. Links and balances all the energy centers.

Tarragon (*Artemisia dracunculus*)
Sixth: Helps us to acknowledge and understand intuitive information that we experience as "gut feelings." Connects us to our inner wisdom.

Tuberose (*Polianthes tuberosa*)
General: Calms and comforts the emotions. Supports healing.
Second: Promotes sensuality and sensitivity. Supports the healing of emotional wounds.
Third: Promotes motivation and enthusiasm.
Fourth: Invites healing love into our lives. Expands our ability to give and receive love. Supports appropriate forgiveness. Promotes trust.
Fifth: Promotes honest, open, and loving communication.
Seventh: Helps in the healing of spiritual injury.

Valerian (*Valeriana officinalis*)
Second: Comforts emotions.
Fourth: Balances the Heart center's emotional responses.
Seventh: Increases love for the Divine.

Verbena, Lemon (*Lippia citriodora*)
General: Clears and cleanses. Clears away negativity.
Second: Promotes healthy emotional boundaries.

Violet (*Viola odorata*)
General: Protects those who are shy or hypersensitive.
Seventh: Increases spirituality in a gentle way for those who have been spiritually injured.

Wormwood (*Artemisia herba alba*)
General: Promotes intuitive dreams and increases intuitive abilities. Eases times of transition.
First, Second, Third: Helps us to deal with fear of death.

Yarrow, Blue (*Achillea millefolium*)
General: Calms and protects.
Third: Promotes courage.
Fourth: Promotes healthy love for oneself and others.
Sixth: Promotes discernment. Promotes intuition, intuitive dreams, and visions.

Appendix II:
Quick Reference to Basic Hand Positions

1 & 2. **Open Toes and Close Toes**

Key purpose: To begin and end a subtle energy therapy session by gently opening and closing the energy centers in order to help balance the subtle anatomy. It links the physical body and subtle anatomy together so subtle energy therapy can work on all levels.

Physical: Balances, helping with any uncomfortable physical state.

Psychological: Balances, helping with any uncomfortable mental or emotional state such as worry, confusion, excessive thoughts, shock, moodiness, or exhausted nerves.

Spiritual: Balances, helping with any spiritual issues.

3. **Forehead Spread**

Key purpose: To balance mental activities and open the receiver to healing energy.

Physical: Useful for relieving headaches, vision problems, and sinus problems.

Psychological: Helps to clear mental confusion, worry, obsessive thoughts, doubt, mental conflict, creative blocks, problems in learning, and apathy.

Spiritual: Helps to establish a connection to a spiritual path. Eases fear, confusion, or anger about religion and/or spirituality. Helps recognition of and response to intuitive information.

4. **Simple Hold**

Key purpose: To bring an area of the body into balance to support the body's natural healing ability.

Physical: Balances, helping with any uncomfortable physical state.

Psychological: Helps any symptom of mental or emotional imbalance such as worry, confusion, excessive thoughts, shock, moodiness, or exhausted nerves.

Spiritual: Helps to initiate and increase spiritual awareness.

5. **Filling**

Key purpose: To increase/restore physical, mental, and emotional vitality.

179

Physical: Helps to relieve exhaustion and fatigue.

Psychological: Helps to ease emotional and mental exhaustion, burn-out, stress, and emotional emptiness.

Spiritual: Gently increases the energy in the subtle bodies.

6 & 7. Combing and Smoothing the Energy Field

Key purpose: To clear, balance, and seal the energy field, especially after a subtle energy therapy session. To promote a general sense of well-being by soothing and comforting the subtle bodies.

Physical: Helps uncomfortable physical states such as sunburn, skin rashes, and agitation due to stress or worry.

Psychological: Eases uncomfortable emotional states such as fear, anger, or grief.

Spiritual: Helps to repair an energy field damaged by physical or emotional trauma. Supports healthy boundaries during times of negative influences from relationships or physical surroundings.

Appendix III:
Suggested Subtle Energy Therapy Sessions
for Common Imbalances

Below are suggestions for subtle energy therapy sessions found to be effective for certain common imbalances. Experiment, practice, and discover how these may be of help to you and to others. You may choose to incorporate both essential oils and color following the guidelines given at the beginning of Chapter 6.

Physical

Backache: Open Toes, Simple Hold (associated energy center or centers and specific area), Close Toes, Comb and Smooth.

Burnout (adrenal support): Open Toes, Forehead Spread, Simple Hold (First energy center and then over both adrenal glands), Filling, Close Toes, Comb and Smooth.

Congestion, respiratory: Open Toes, Simple Hold (Fourth energy center then lung area), Close Toes, Comb and Smooth.

Disorientation (following physical trauma): Open and Close Toes, Forehead Spread, Close Toes, Comb and Smooth.

Ear, ache: Open Toes, Simple Hold (Fifth energy center then over the ears), Close Toes, Comb and Smooth.

Fatigue: Open Toes, Forehead Spread, Filling, Close Toes, Comb and Smooth.

Feet, sore: Open Toes, Simple Hold (tops then bottoms of feet), Close Toes, Comb and Smooth.

Headache: (Do not use for migraines.) Open Toes, Forehead Spread, Close Toes, Comb and Smooth.

Indigestion: Open Toes, Simple Hold (Third energy center then stomach area), Close Toes, Comb and Smooth.

Legs, poor circulation: Open Toes, Simple Hold (First energy center then both legs), Filling, Close Toes, Comb and Smooth.

Muscle, ache: Open Toes, Simple Hold (specific area), Close Toes, Comb and Smooth.

Travel (Motion) Sickness: Open Toes, Simple Hold (First energy center then Third energy center), Forehead Spread (if head is affected), Close Toes, Comb and Smooth.

<u>Vision problems:</u> Open Toes, Forehead Spread, Close Toes, Comb and Smooth.

Psychological

<u>Anger:</u> Open Toes, Simple Hold (Third energy center then Fourth energy center), Close Toes, Comb and Smooth.

<u>Anxiety:</u> Open Toes, Simple Hold (Second energy center), Forehead Spread, Close Toes, Comb and Smooth.

<u>Creative Blocks:</u> Open Toes, Simple Hold (Second energy center, then Fifth energy center, then Sixth energy center), Close Toes, Comb and Smooth.

<u>Disorientation (following mental or emotional trauma):</u> Open Toes, Simple Hold (Feet energy centers), Forehead Spread, Close Toes, Comb and Smooth.

<u>Emotions, unreleased:</u> Open Toes, Simple Hold (Second energy center), Close Toes, Comb and Smooth.

<u>Fear:</u> Open Toes, Simple Hold (Second energy center then Third energy center), Close Toes, Comb and Smooth.

<u>Grief:</u> Open Toes, Simple Hold (Fourth energy center), Close Toes, Comb and Smooth.

<u>Insecure (feeling unsafe):</u> Open Toes, Simple Hold (First energy center holding hands six inches above the body and then Feet energy centers), Close Toes, Comb and Smooth.

<u>Irritability:</u> Open Toes, Simple Hold (Third energy center), Forehead Spread, Close Toes, Comb and Smooth.

<u>Mental Fog:</u> Open Toes, Forehead Spread, Simple Hold (Feet energy centers), Close Toes, Comb and Smooth.

<u>Memory, poor:</u> Open Toes, Forehead Spread, Close Toes, Comb and Smooth.

<u>Sorrow:</u> Open Toes, Simple Hold (Fourth energy center), Close Toes, Comb and Smooth.

<u>Sleep, poor, if related to thoughts and/or emotions:</u> Open Toes, Forehead Spread, Simple Hold (Second energy center then Fourth energy center), Close Toes, Comb and Smooth.

<u>Stress, general:</u> Open Toes, Forehead Spread, Simple Hold (Fourth energy center), Close Toes, Comb and Smooth.

<u>Thoughts, obsessive:</u> Open Toes, Forehead Spread, Simple Hold (Second energy center then Fourth energy center), Close Toes, Comb and Smooth.

Thoughts, rigid: Open Toes, Forehead Spread, Simple Hold (First energy center then Fourth energy center), Close Toes, Comb and Smooth.

Thoughts, unreleased: Open Toes, Forehead Spread, Close Toes, Comb and Smooth.

Worry, obsessive: Open Toes, Forehead Spread, Simple Hold (Second energy center, then Third energy center, then Fourth energy center), Close Toes, Comb and Smooth.

Spiritual

Congestion, in the subtle bodies (all levels): Open Toes, Forehead Spread, Simple Hold (First through Fifth energy centers for one minute each), Close Toes, Comb and Smooth.

Disconnection, logical mind from spiritual perspective: Open Toes, Forehead Spread, Simple Hold (Sixth energy center with hands on either side of the head over ears), Close Toes, Comb and Smooth.

Disconnection, spirit from body: Open Toes, Forehead Spread, Simple Hold (Fourth energy center, then legs, then feet), Close Toes, Comb and Smooth.

Imbalance, between intuitive and rational mind: Open Toes, Forehead Spread, Close Toes, Comb and Smooth.

Spirituality, blocked (spiritual energy cannot enter): Open Toes, Forehead Spread, Simple Hold (Fifth energy center), Close Toes, Comb and Smooth.

Spirituality, rigid (spiritual energy is not flexible): Open Toes, Forehead Spread, Simple Hold (Heart energy center), Close Toes, Comb and Smooth.

Appendix IV:
"Listening to an Essential Oil"
Exercise Fill-in Form

Chapter 3 discusses how the subtle properties of essential oils are determined, and includes an exercise called "Listening to an Essential Oil." For your convenience, make a copy of this fill-in form and use it when practicing this exercise.

Holding the Oil:
    Color:
    Feeling:
    Memory:
    Texture:
    Sound:
    Aroma: (May be different than the oil itself.)

Smelling the Oil:
    Do you like or dislike the aroma?
    Is there any place or places in your body that are affected by this fragrance?
    Is there an energy center that is touched or stimulated?
    Does it make you feel relaxed or energized?
    Do you receive any sense impressions?
        Color:
        Shape:
        Temperature:
        Texture:
        Image:
        Sound:
        Memory:

A "Conversation"
The responses may come in any sense—words, feelings, images, or sounds.
    What are your subtle properties?
    What energy center are you most connected with?
    What are your gifts for subtle energy therapy?
    What are your spiritual gifts?
    Is there anything about you that you want me to know?
    Is there anything you want to communicate to me now?

Appendix V:
Quick Reference to Key Essential Oils Used
for Subtle Energy Therapy

The following essential oils are those mentioned in Chapter 3 as the Basic, Intermediate, and Advanced Oils used in subtle energy therapy. They are listed here in alphabetical order, not in order of importance.

Angelica: Grounds. Connects us with the angelic realm. Strengthens spirituality.

Bay Laurel: Clears and cleanses the energy centers. Opens the mind. Promotes intuition.

Benzoin: Grounds. Strengthens and comforts. Steadies and focuses the mind, especially for meditation or prayer.

Bergamot: Clears and cleanses. Brings in positive, optimistic energy. Uplifts yet calms. Eases wounds of the heart, especially grief.

Cardamom: Promotes generosity and graciousness with others. Warms the emotions. Promotes creativity and sensuality.

Cedarwood: Clears and cleanses. Strengthens and balances. Steadies the mind and promotes the ability to concentrate.

Chamomile German: Calms and comforts, especially the emotions. Supports calm, gentle verbal communication.

Chamomile Roman: Calms and comforts, especially the emotions. Supports calm, gentle verbal communication.

Clary Sage: Calms, uplifts, restores, and inspires. Supports intuition.

Coriander: Promotes enthusiasm, optimism, and creativity. Promotes emotional warmth.

Elemi: Grounds. Helps to calm, strengthen, and balance. Opens the mind to mystical experiences.

Eucalyptus: Clears and cleanses. Helps to clear energy blocks and negative energy. Inspires. Promotes mental clarity and positivity.

Frankincense: Grounds. Calms and comforts. Stabilizes emotions. Expands the subtle bodies. Focuses and strengthens spirituality.

Geranium: Helps to calm and balance the emotions. Has a nurturing quality. Promotes feminine creativity.

Grapefruit: Clears negative energy blocks. Uplifts and promotes optimism. Promotes intuition and mental clarity. Refreshes the mind.

Helichrysum: Clears energy blocks caused by challenging emotions. Helps to let go of emotional wounds and promotes acceptance.

Jasmine: Calms and uplifts. Unites and harmonizes to promote wholeness. Promotes creative and artistic development. Promotes sensitivity and sensuality.

Juniper: Clears negative energy and uplifts. Clears energy blocks in the subtle bodies. Protects against negative influences, especially from other people.

Lavender: One of the most important subtle energy essential oils. Balances and integrates all energy centers and subtle bodies. Brings in positive energy. Useful in all energy healing techniques to cleanse, clear, calm, and balance (gently energizes or gently relaxes). Promotes compassion, forgiveness, and acceptance.

Lemon: Clears and cleanses. Clarifies, uplifts, and invigorates. Promotes mental vitality.

Marjoram: Comforts and calms. Warms. Promotes sincerity and the ability to give. Helps to accept emotional loss.

Melissa: Comforts and uplifts. Promotes understanding, acceptance, and a sense of peace.

Myrrh: Grounds, warms, and strengthens. Helps us to let go of the past and move forward. Strengthens spirituality.

Neroli: Brings positive energy. Calms and uplifts. Eases grief and sorrow. Links lower and higher energy centers—body and spirit.

Oakmoss: Grounds. Promotes a sense of security.

Orange: Brings in joyful, positive energy. Uplifts. Gently clears energy blocks. Promotes joy in relationships.

Palmarosa: Calms. Supports all levels of healing—physical, emotional, mental, and spiritual. Promotes self-acceptance and personal growth.

Patchouli: Grounds and stabilizes. Strengthens and rejuvenates. Calms and promotes a sense of peace. Promotes creativity.

Peppermint: Uplifts, awakens, and revitalizes. Stimulates the conscious mind. Promotes clear perception.

Rose: Brings in positive energy, especially love and compassion. Promotes a sense of well-being. Helps to fill holes in the subtle bodies. Promotes hope, acceptance, and patience. Eases and comforts heartaches.

Rosemary: Clears and cleanses. Strengthens, energizes, and motivates. Clears and energizes the mind.

<u>Rosewood:</u> Grounds. Brings in calm, positive energy. Clears energy blocks. Gently opens us to spirituality.

<u>Sandalwood:</u> Grounds. Calms and comforts. Supports healing on all levels—physical, emotional, mental, spiritual. Supports spiritual development. Promotes a sense of peace.

<u>Spruce:</u> Clears, cleanses, and rejuvenates. Supports intuition and encourages new insights.

<u>Thyme:</u> Clears energy blocks. Strengthens and energizes. Promotes self-confidence, personal strength, and courage. Motivates.

<u>Vetiver:</u> Grounds, strengthens, stabilizes, calms, and protects. Promotes a deep sense of belonging.

Appendix VI:
Quick Reference to Key Essential Oils to Use During a Subtle Energy Therapy Session

The following are some of the ways essential oils are used during a subtle energy session. This is not an exhaustive list as there are many more applications and additional oils that could be used. The information here is to provide a quick reference for the most common applications and the essential oils associated with those applications. See Chapter 4, under "Applications for Using Essential Oils for Subtle Energy Therapy," #4, "Working with the Energy Centers" for directions to make misters and anointing oils. For more information about the individual essential oils and how they relate to the energy centers, refer to Chapters 3 and 4.

To clear and cleanse the room and/or yourself:
Use in a diffuser or mister in the area before and after working with subtle energy therapy.
Clearing and cleansing is a part of "Setting Sacred Space." See Chapter 4 for more information.
Bergamot, Cedarwood, Eucalyptus, Lemon, Lemongrass, Lime, Pine, Rosemary, Spruce.

To bring in positive energy:
Use in a diffuser or mister in the area before working with subtle energy therapy.
Bringing in positive energy is a part of "Setting Sacred Space." See Chapter 4 for more information.
Basil, Bergamot, Cedarwood, Eucalyptus, Lavender, Neroli, Orange, Petitgrain, Rose, Rosewood.

Blends to both cleanse the room and bring in positive energy:
Use in a diffuser or mister in the area before and after working with subtle energy therapy.
Clearing and cleansing and bringing in positive energy are parts of "Setting Sacred Space." See Chapter 4 for more information.
Lavender/Cedarwood/Orange, Lemon/Orange, Pine/Rosewood, Bergamot/Lavender.

To set up boundaries to provide protection to the area:
Use in a diffuser or mister in the area, or at the perimeter of the area before working with subtle energy therapy.
Setting up or establishing boundaries are a part of "Setting Sacred Space." See Chapter 4 for more information.
Fennel, Lemongrass, Oakmoss, Peppermint, Rosemary.

To ask for spiritual and/or angelic guidance:
Use as an anointing oil on the Sixth and Seventh energy centers before working with subtle energy therapy.
Angelica Root, Bay Laurel, Black Pepper, Cedarwood, Cypress, Frankincense, Jasmine, Lemon, Neroli, Orange, Rose, Rosemary.

Blends to link the Hands centers to the Heart center:
Use as an anointing oil on the Hands and Heart centers before working with subtle energy therapy.
Lavender/Rose, Bergamot/Rose, Cardamom/Bergamot, Chamomile Roman/Sandalwood, Helichrysum/Geranium, Geranium/Frankincense.

To promote the healing capability in your hands:
Use as an anointing oil on the palms of each of your hands before working with subtle energy therapy.
Bergamot, Cardamom, Chamomile German or Roman, Geranium, Helichrysum, Lavender, Orange, Rose, Rosewood, Sandalwood.

To ground yourself and/or your receiver:
Use as an anointing oil on the Feet centers before or after working with subtle energy therapy.
Cedarwood, Frankincense, Myrrh, Oakmoss, Patchouli, Rosewood, Sandalwood, Vetiver.

To help clear away energy blocks:
Use as a mist on the energy field or as an anointing oil on specific energy centers while working with subtle energy therapy.
Black Pepper, Eucalyptus, Fir Douglas, Grapefruit, Helichyrsum, Juniper, Lemon, Melissa, Orange, Rosewood, Thyme.

To quiet the mind to better receive healing energy:
Use in a diffuser, as a mist, or as an anointing oil before working with subtle energy therapy.
Bergamot, Cedarwood, Frankincense, Marjoram, Sandalwood.

To assist the First (Root) energy center:
Use as a mist or anointing oil on or over this center before and/or during working with subtle energy therapy.
Cedarwood, Frankincense, Myrrh, Oakmoss, Patchouli, Rosewood, Sandalwood, Vetiver.

To assist the Second (Sacral) energy center:
Use as a mist or anointing oil on or over this center before and/or during working with subtle energy therapy.
Cardamon, Coriander, Dill, Geranium, Jasmine, Juniper, Nutmeg, Orange, Rose, Ylang Ylang.

To assist the Third (Solar Plexus) energy center:
Use as a mist or anointing oil on or over this center before and/or during working with subtle energy therapy.
Black Pepper, Clove, Fennel, Ginger, Palmarosa, Peppermint, Petitgrain, Pine, Rosemary, Tea Tree, Thyme.

To assist the Fourth (Heart) energy center:
Use as a mist or anointing oil on or over this center before and/or during working with subtle energy therapy.
Bergamot, Helichrysum, Jasmine, Lavender, Mandarin, Marjoram, Melissa, Neroli, Orange, Rose.

To assist the Fifth (Throat) energy center:
Use as a mist or anointing oil on or over this center before and/or during working with subtle energy therapy.
Bergamot, Chamomile German or Roman, Lavender, Lemon, Orange, Peppermint, Sandalwood.

To assist the Sixth (Brow) energy center:
Use as a mist or anointing oil on or over this center before and/or during working with subtle energy therapy.

Anise, Basil, Bay Laurel, Benzoin, Cedarwood, Clary Sage, Elemi, Eucalyptus, Fir, Frankincense, Grapefruit, Jasmine, Lemon, Lemongrass, Peppermint, Rosemary, Spruce.

To assist the Seventh (Crown) energy center:
Use as a mist or anointing oil on or over this center before and/or during working with subtle energy therapy.
Angelica, Cedarwood, Elemi, Frankincense, Lavender, Myrrh, Neroli, Orange, Rose, Rosewood, Sandalwood.

To assist the Hands energy centers:
Use as a mist or anointing oil on or over this center before and/or during working with subtle energy therapy.
Bergamot, Cardamom, Chamomile German or Roman, Geranium, Helichrysum, Lavender, Orange, Rose, Rosewood.

To assist the Feet energy centers:
Use as a mist or anointing oil on or over this center before and/or during working with subtle energy therapy.
Benzoin, Cedarwood, Frankincense, Myrrh, Oakmoss, Patchouli, Rosewood, Sandalwood, Vetiver.

Recommended Reading by Chapters

Chapter 1: Introduction to Aromatherapy
The History of Aromatherapy
The Nature of Essential Oils
How Essential Oils Affect Us
Methods of Using Essential Oils
Essential Oil Safety

The Healing Intelligence of Essential Oils by Kurt Schnaubelt
Aromatherapy: A Complete Guide to the Healing Art, Second Edition, by Kathi Keville and Mindy Green
Practical Aromatherapy for Self-Care by Joni Keim
Aromatherapy: A Lifetime Guide to Healing with Essential Oils by Valerie Gennari Cooksley
Aromatherapy for Dummies by Kathy Keville
The Directory of Essential Oils by Wanda Sellar
Aromatherapy for the Healthy Child by Valerie Ann Worwood
Aromatherapy for Massage Practitioners by Ingrid Martin
Subtle Aromatherapy by Patricia Davis
Aromatherapy for Healing the Spirit by Gabriel Mojay

Chapter 2: Introduction to Subtle Energy Therapy
Examples of Subtle Energy Therapies
Our Energy Anatomy
The Healing Nature of Compassionate Touch
Preparing Your Hands and Yourself
Exercises with Subtle Energy
Using Intention and Visualization for Subtle Energy Therapy
Using Color for Subtle Energy Therapy
The Role of Intuition
Subtle Energy Terminology

Eastern Body, Western Mind by Anodea Judith
The Sevenfold Journey by Anodea Judith and Selene Vega
Chakra Balancing by Anodea Judith
Anatomy of the Spirit by Carolyn Myss
Wheels of Light by Roselyn Bruyere

Hands of Light by Barbara Ann Brennan
Vibrational Medicine by Richard Gerber, M. D.
Hands-on Healing by Jack Angelo
Your Hands Can Heal by Ric A. Weinman
You Already Know What to Do by Sharon Franquemont

Chapter 3: The Subtle Properties of Essential Oils
What is Vibrational Medicine?
How the Subtle Properties of Essential Oils Are Determined
"Listening to an Essential Oil" Exercise
The Subtle Properties of Essential Oils: A-Z
Choosing Your First Essential Oils

Aromatherapy for Healing the Spirit by Gabriel Mojay
Subtle Aromatherapy by Patricia Davis
Vibrational Medicine by Richard Gerber, M. D.
Aromatherapy Anointing Oils by Joni Keim and Ruah Bull
Daily Aromatherapy by Joni Keim and Ruah Bull
The Fragrant Heavens by Valerie Ann Worwood
The Blossoming Heart by Robbi Zeck, ND

Chapter 4: Using Essential Oils for Subtle Energy Therapy
Using Essential Oils with Intention
Methods of Using Essential Oils for Subtle Energy Therapy
Applications for Using Essential Oils for Subtle Energy Therapy
Essential Oils for the Energy Centers

Sacred Space: Clearing and Enhancing the Energy of Your Home by Denise Linn
Aromatherapy for Healing the Spirit by Gabriel Mojay
Subtle Aromatherapy by Patricia Davis
Vibrational Medicine by Richard Gerber, M. D.
Aromatherapy Anointing Oils by Joni Keim and Ruah Bull
Daily Aromatherapy by Joni Keim and Ruah Bull
The Fragrant Heavens by Valerie Ann Worwood
The Blossoming Heart by Robbi Zeck, ND
The Sevenfold Journey by Anodea Judith and Selene Vega
Anatomy of the Spirit by Carolyn Myss
Wheels of Light by Roselyn Bruyere

Chapter 5: Helping Ourselves
Self-care Questionnaire
The Four Dimensions of Well-Being
Self-care Exercise
Stress: A Part of Life
Stress Reduction and Management
Emotions Associated with the Energy Centers
Assessing Your Energy Centers
Balancing Your Energy Centers and Subtle Bodies

Hypnosis for Change by Josie Hadley and Carol Staudacher
Buffalo Woman Comes Singing by Brooke Medicine Eagle
Subtle Energy by William Collinge, Ph.D.
Sevenfold Journey by Anodea Judith & Selene Vega
Pendulum Power, Greg Neilsen and Joseph Polansky
Affirmations by Cathy Guiswite

Chapter 6: Helping Others
Ethical Responsibility
Active Listening
Basic Hand Positions to Use for Subtle Energy Therapy
Giving a Subtle Energy Therapy Session
Ending a Subtle Energy Therapy Session
After a Subtle Energy Therapy Session
Case Studies with Ruah Bull
An Exercise with a Hand Position and an Essential Oil

How Can I Help? Stories and Reflections on Service by Ram Dass
Compassion in Action by Ram Dass
The Ethics of Caring by Kylea Taylor
Energy Medicine by Donna Eden
Hands of Life by Julie Motz
A Handbook for Light Workers by David Cousins
Healing Words by Larry Dossey

Bibliography

A Gift for Healing, Deborah Cowens (New York: Crown Trade Paperbacks, 1996).

A Handbook for Light Workers, David Cousins (Dartmouth, England: Barton House, 1993).

Accepting Your Power to Heal: The Personal Practice of Therapeutic Touch, Dolores Kreiger, Ph.D. (Santa Fe, NM: Bear and Company Publications, 1993).

Affirmations, Cathy Guiswite (New York: Andrews and McMeel, 1996).

Anatomy of the Spirit, Carolyn Myss (New York: Harmony Books, 1996.)

Aromatherapy: A Complete Guide to the Healing Art, Kathy Keville and Mindy Green (Freedom, CA: The Crossing Press, 1995).

Aromatherapy for Vibrant Health and Beauty, Roberta Wilson (Garden City Park, NY: Avery Publishing Group, 1995).

Aromatherapy for Healing the Spirit, Gabriel Mojay (New York: Henry Holt and Company, 1996).

Aromatherapy: Scent and Psyche, Peter Damian and Kate Damian (Rochester, VT: Healing Arts Press, 1991).

Buffalo Woman Comes Singing, Brooke Medicine Eagle (New York: Ballantine Books, 1991).

Aromatherapy: A Lifetime Guide to Healing with Essential Oils, Valerie Gennari Cooksley (Englewood Cliffs, NJ: Prentice Hall, 1996).

Compassion in Action, Ram Dass (New York: Harper and Row, 1998).

Creative Visualization, Shakti Gawain (Berkeley, CA: Whatever Publishing, 1978).

Eastern Body, Western Mind, Anodea Judith (New York: Harper and Row, 1998).

Energy Medicine, Donna Eden (New York: Tarcher/Putnam, 1998).

Empowerment Through Reiki, Paula Horan (Twin Lakes, WI: Lotus Light Publications, 1990).

Full Catastrophe Living, Jon Kabat-Zinn, Ph.D. (New York: Dell Publishing, 1990).

Hands of Life, Julie Motz (New York: Bantam Books, 1998).

Hands-On Healing, Jack Angelo (Rochester, VT: Healing Arts Press, 1997).

Healers on Healing, Edited by Richard Carlson (New York: Tarcher Putnam, 1995).

Healing with Love, Leonard Laskow, M.D. (New York: Harper Collins, 1992).

Healing Words, Larry Dossey (New York: Harper-Collins, 1993).

How Can I Help? Stories and Reflections on Service, Ram Dass (New York: Knopf Publishing, 1985).

Hypnosis for Change, Josie Hadley and Carol Staudacher (Oakland, CA: New Harbinger Publishing, 1991).

Infinite Mind, Valerie V. Hunt (Malibu, CA: Malibu Publications, 1989).

Inner Knowing, Edited by Helen Palmer (New York: Tarcher Putnam, 1998).

Magical Aromatherapy, Scott Cunningham (St. Paul, MN: Llewellan Publishing, 1995).

Pendulum Power, Greg Neilsen and Joseph Polansky (New York: Harper Collins, 1987).

Psychic Protection, William Bloom (New York: Simon and Schuster, 1996).

Sacred Space: Clearing and Enhancing the Energy of Your Home, Denise Linn (New York: Ballantine Books, 1995).

Sevenfold Journey, Anodeath Judith and Selene Vega (Freedom, CA: Crossing Press, 1993).

Spiritual Cleaning, Draja Mickaharic (York Beach, ME: Samuel Weiser, Inc., 1982).

The Chakras and the Human Energy Field, S. Karcgulla and D. Kunz (Wheaton, IL: Theosophical Publishing House, 1976).

The Essence of Magic, Mary K. Greer (Van Nuys, CA: Newcastle Publishing, 1993).

The Ethics of Caring, Kylea Taylor (New York: Hanford Mead Publishing, 1995).

The Healing Energy of Your Hands, Michael Bradford (Freedom, CA: The Crossing Press, 1993).

The Healing Power of Aromatherapy, Hasnain Walji, Ph. D. (Rocklin, CA: Prima Publishing, 1996).

The Illustrated Encyclopedia of Essential Oils, Julia Lawless (Rockport, MA: Element Books, 1995).

The Inward Arc, Frances Vaughan (Nevada City, CA: Blue Dolphin Publishing, Inc., 1995).

The Light Inside the Dark, John Tarrant (New York: Harper Collins, 1998).

The Personal Aura, D. Kunz (Wheaton, IL: Theosophical Publishing House, 1991).

The Pendulum Kit, Sig Longren (New York: Fireside Books, 1990).

The World of Aromatherapy, Edited by Jeanne Rose and Susan Earle (Berkeley, CA: Frog, Ltd., 1996).

Subtle Aromatherapy, Patricia Davis (England: C. W. Daniel Company Limited, 1991).

Subtle Energy, William Collinge, Ph.D. (New York: Warner Books, 1998).

Vibrational Medicine, Dr. Richard Gerber (Santa Fe, NM: Bear and Company Publications, 1988).

Wheels of Light, Rosalyn Bruyere (New York: Fireside, 1994).

Wheels of Life, Anodea Judith (St. Paul, MN: Llewellyn Publications, 1996).

Your Hands Can Heal, Ric A. Weinman (New York: Penguin Books, 1992).

Your Healing Hands, Richard Gordon (Berkeley, CA: Wingbow Press, 1978).

INDEX

A

Active listening, 144
Affecting consciousness, 70
Affirmations, 2, 55, 58, **132**, 135, 137
Aldehydes, 6
Ammi Visnaga, 169
Amygdala, 6
Amyris, 169
Angelica
  as advanced essential oil, 63
  for Seventh energy center, 94, 194
  for Forehead Spread, 148
  for spiritual guidance, 69
  quick reference, 187
  subtle properties of, 38
Anise
  for Sixth energy center, 91, 194
  subtle properties of, 38
Anointing
  definition of, 66
  to work with energy centers, 72
Anointing oil
  to give to receiver, 163
  to make, 66
Archier, Micheline, 3
Aroma. See also smell, sense of
  pathway of, 5
  perception of, 6
  reception of, 5
  transmission of, 5
Aromatherapy. See also essential oils
  cosmetic, 1
  definition of, 1
  historic use of, xvi
  history of, 2
  medical, 1
  psychological, 1
  subtle, 2
Artemisia, 169
Ask for spiritual guidance, 69
  quick reference, 192
Assessing your energy centers, 121
Astral body, **19**, 170, 172
Azalea, 170

B

Balancing an energy center, definition, 30
Balancing your energy centers
    & subtle bodies, 126
Basic hand positions, 145-155
Basil, 39
Bath, 7
  for stress relief, 118
Bay Laurel, 39
Bearheart, Margo, 12
Benzoin
  as advanced essential oil, 63
  quick reference, 187
  subtle properties of, 39
Bergamot
  for affecting consciousness, 71
  as basic essential oil, 62
  to bring in positive energy, 191
  quick reference, 187
  for positive energy, 68
  for stress relief, 118
  subtle properties of, 40
Birch, 170
Black Pepper, 40
Body language, 144
Body mister, 8
  for stress relief, 119
Boundaries
  essential oils, to set up, 69
  "healthy", definition, 31
  respecting personal,143
  to set up, 69
  quick reference to set up, 192
Boundary blends, 69
Breath, Center in Your, 22
Breath Meditation, 117
Breathing exercises, 117
Brennan, Barbara, 11
Broom, 170
Bruyere, Rosalyn, 11
Bucco Leaves, 170
Bull, Ruah
  case studies, 164
  earth energy healing quote, 12

C

Cabreuva, 170
Calamus, 170
Cajeput, 170
Cardamom
  as advanced essential oil, 63
  subtle properties of, 41
  quick reference, 187
Carvi, 170
Cascarilla, 171
Case studies, 164
Cedarwood
  for affecting consciousness, 71
  as basic essential oil, 62
  for clearing and cleansing, 68
  for Forehead Spread technique, 148
  for guidance, 192
  for positive energy, 68, 191
  quick reference, 187
  subtle properties of, 41
Cedrella, 171
Center in Your Breath exercise, 22
Chakras, 13. See energy centers
Chamomile, German
  in baths, 7
  color of, 34
  in cosmetic applications, 1
  for Forehead Spread technique, 157
  as intermediate essential oil, 62
  for Open Toes/Close Toes
    technique, 147
  quick reference, 187
  subtle properties of, 41
Chamomile Roman
  as basic essential oil, 62
  in baths, 7
  in cosmetic applications, 1
  for Open Toes/Close Toes
    technique, 147
  quick reference, 187
  for stress relief, 118
  subtle properties of, 42
Champaca, 171
Choosing your first essential oils, 61
Cinnamon, Leaf, 42
Cistus, 171
Citronella, 43

Clary Sage
  as intermediate essential oil, 62
  in baths, 7
  plant gestures of, 34
  quick reference, 187
  for stress relief, 118
  subtle properties of, 43
Clear and cleanse, 68
  quick reference, 191
Clear energy blocks, quick reference, 192
Clearing and cleansing blends, 68
Clove, 44
Color
  associated with energy centers, 15-18
  blue, indigo, 29
  blue, sky, 29
  for Combing & Smoothing
    technique, 154
  essential oils', 3
  for Filling technique, 153
  for Forehead Spread technique, 148
  green, 29
  green, dark, moss, 29
  gold, 29
  for Open Toes/Close Toes
    technique, 147
  as plant gesture and signature, 34
  for Simple Hold technique, 139
  orange, 28
  pink, 29
  red, 28
  subtle bodies change, 13
  for subtle energy therapy, 28
  violet, 29
  white, 29
  yellow, 29
Combing & Smoothing technique, 153
  aromatherapy, subtle, for, 155
  quick reference, 180
  visualization & color exercise for, 154
Communication, positive,
  session for, 161
Compassionate touch,
  healing nature of, 20
Compress, 8
Confidence, session for, 160
Confidentiality, 143

Consciousness, affecting, 71
Copaiva Balm, 171
Coriander
    as advanced essential oil, 63
    quick reference, 187
    subtle properties of, 44
Cortisol, 115
Costus Root, 171
Cowens, Deborah, 21
Creativity, enhancing, session for, 159
Croton Anisatum, 171
Curry Leaves, 171
Cypress, 44
Cypriol, 172

D

Davis, Calvin, 11
Davis, Patricia, 33
Daydreams, helpful, 129
Dead Sea Scrolls, 20
Diet, 108
Diffusers, 5, **7**, **66**, 67
Dill, 45
Dis-ease, 20
Dis-stress, 115
Dossey, Larry, 65

E

Earth Energy Healing, 12
Edwards, Victoria, 3
Elecampane, 172
Elemi
    as advanced essential oil, 63
    for Forehead Spread, 149
    for Open Toes/Close Toes, 147
    quick reference, 187
    subtle properties of, 45
Emotional body, 19. See also Astral Body
Emotional well-being, 111.
        See also Feelings
Emotions, associated with energy
    centers, 119
Empathy, misplaced, 144
Energizing, session for, 157
Energy anatomy, 13-20
Energy centers (chakras).
        See also individual energy centers
    assessing your, 121

assessing with pendulum, 125
balanced state, 14
"balancing", definition, 30
color and, 15-18
congested feelings
        associated with, 73-101
"connecting with", definition, 31
constricted feelings
        associated with, 73-101
emotions associated with, 119
essential oils for, 73-104
explanation of each, 13-18
Feet, 18
Fifth, 17
First, 15
Fourth, 16
function of, 13
Hands, 18
imbalances or blockages in, 73-101
"linking", definition, 31
location of, 15-18
meditation exercise, 25
primary, 14
questionnaire, 121
reaction to stress, 14
Second, 15
secondary, 14
Seventh, 17
Sixth, 17
special technique to tend to, 136
spin of, 13
strengthening, 134
subtle bodies and, 13, 18-20
Third, 16
working with, 72
Energy Center Meditation, 25
Energy exercises, 24-27
Energy field, 11, 12, **13**, 18, 31, 153,
        170, 171. See also subtle bodies
Energy workouts, 136
Epilepsy, 9
Erigeron, 172
Eriocephalus, 172
Essenes, 20
Essential oils. See also individual oils
    to affect consciousness, 71
    applications for subtle
        energy therapy, 67

chemical make-up of, 6
choosing your first, 61
to clear and cleanse, 67
cosmetic uses of, 1
determining subtle properties of, 33
dilutions, 8
effects on the body from, 1
for energy centers, 73-104
energy nature of, 33
extraction of, 4
factors for quality, 3
from plant parts, 4
how subtle properties
    are determined, 33
how to store, 9
how we are affected by, 5
indicators of subtle properties, 34
"Listening to the Oils" exercise, 35
medical uses of, 1
methods of using, 5, **6-8**, **66**,
nature of, 3
not "oily", 3
pathway of their aroma, 5
plant parts used for, 4
for positive energy, 68
properties of, 1
price of, 4
psychological uses of, 1
quality of, 3
quick reference to, 187
for setting up boundaries, 69
safety, guidelines, 8-10
subtle properties of, 37-62
sources of, 3
top 12 advanced, 63
top 12 basic, 62
top 12 intermediate, 62
traditional use of subtle properties, 33
for spiritual guidance, 70
for subtle energy therapy, 65
for transformative techniques, 2
using with intention, 27, 35
viscosities, 3
volatility of, 3
Esters, 6
Estibany, Oskar, 65
Etheric body, **19**, 25
Ethical responsibility, 143

Eucalyptus
    for affecting consciousness, 71
    as basic essential oil, 62
    in baths, 7
    for clearing and cleansing, 68
    in medical applications, 1
    quick reference, 187
    subtle properties of, 46
Eustress, 115
Exercise, physical, 19, **108**
Exercises. See also individual techniques
    Activate Your Hands, 23
    Appreciate Your Hands, 22
    balancing energy centers
        and subtle bodies 126-141
    Being Present, 132
    breathing, 117
    Center in Your Breath, 22
    creating, 129
    Energy Center Meditation, 25
    experimenting with hand positions
        and essential oils, 166
    Feeling Subtle Energy with
        Your Hands, 24
    Four Dimensions, 126
    Helpful Daydreams, 129
    Helping Hand, 137
    "Listening to the Oils," 35
    Nourishment Through the
        Senses, 130
    Preparing Your Hands, 21-23
    self-care activities, 105-107,
        113, 121, 126-141
    sensing the subtle bodies, 24
    to strengthen energy centers, 134
    Taking Time/Making Time, 127
    Tending to an Energy Center, 136
    Tending Touch, 136

F
Feelings, 2, 14, 19, 37, 106, 112, **119**,
    137. See also Emotional well-being
Feeling Subtle Energy with
    Your Hands, 24
Feet energy centers
    affirmations for, 134
    to assist, quick reference, 194
    blends, 102

color and, 18, 29
essential oils for, 100
explanation of, 18
imbalances in, 101
strengthening, 135
questions to assess, 124
Fennel, 46
Filling technique
Aromatherapy, subtle, for, 153
energizing technique, 153
quick reference, 179
visualization & color exercise for, 153
Fifth energy center (Throat)
affirmations for, 133
to assist, quick reference, 193
blends, 88-90
color and, 17, 29
essential oils for, 87
explanation of, 17
imbalances in, 88
strengthening, 135
questions to assess, 123
Fir, Douglas, 46
First energy center (Root/Base)
affirmations for, 133
to assist, quick reference, 193
blends, 75
color and, 15, 28
essential oils for, 73-75
explanation of, 15
imbalances in, 74
spin, 14
strengthening, 134
questions to assess, 121
Fitzgerald, Jan, 12
Fokienia, 172
Forehead Spread technique, 148
aromatherapy, subtle, for, 148
quick reference, 179
visualization & color exercise for, 148
Four Dimensions of Well-being, 107-113
Fourth energy center (Heart)
affirmations for, 133
to assist, quick reference, 193
blends, 85
color and, 16, 29
essential oils for, 84

explanation of, 16
imbalances in, 85
strengthening, 135
questions to assess, 122
Frangipani, 172
Frankincense
for affecting consciousness, 71
in baths, 7
as basic essential oil, 62
history of, 34
quick reference, 187
safety of, 8
for stress relief, 118
subtle properties of, 47

G

Galbanum, 172
Galgant Root, 173
Gattefosse, R. M., 2
Gawain, Shakti, 27
Geranium
in cosmetic applications, 1
for creativity, 130
as intermediate essential oil, 63
quick reference, 187
subtle properties of, 47
Gerber, Richard, 18
Ginger, 48
Gingerlily, 173
Ginkel, Betsy, 12
Giving advice, 145
Golden Rod, 173
Grapefruit
for affecting consciousness, 71
as intermediate essential oil, 63
quick reference, 187
subtle properties of, 48
Greenland Moss, 173
Ground yourself and receiver,
quick reference, 192
"Grounded," definition of, 30
Guaiac Wood, 173
Guidance blend, 70
Gurjum, 173

H

Hands
  activate your, 23
  appreciate your, 22
  basic positions, 145
  description of abilities, 21
  feelings subtle energy with, 24
  form of healing, 21
  preparing, 21-23
  to promote healing capability,
      quick reference, 192
Hands energy center
  affirmations for, 134
  to assist, quick reference, 194
  blends, 99
  color and, 18, 29
  essential oils for, 97
  explanation of, 18
  imbalances in, 98
  strengthening, 135
  questions to assess, 124
Hay, 173
Healing, true meaning, xvi
Helichrysum
  as advanced essential oil, 63
  for Forehead Spread technique, 149
  quick reference, 188
  subtle properties of, 49
  to support creativity, 130
Hearing, sense of, 131
Heart conditions, 9
Homeopathic, 9
Hypothalamus, 6
Hyssop, 173

I

Inhalation
  hot water inhalation, 7
  via diffuser, 7
  direct, 7
  pathway, 5, 7
  for stress relief, 118
  via room spray, 7
  working with energy centers, 73
Intention, 27, **65**
Intuition, 13, **29**, 35.
      See Sixth energy center

J

Jasmine
  as intermediate essential oil, 63
  to nurture skin, 130
  quick reference, 188
  subtle properties of, 49
  to support creativity, 129
  for worry, 138
Joyful heart, session for, 160
Judgment, avoiding, 37, 143
Judith, Anodea, 13
Juniper
  to clear and cleanse, 68
  for energy boundaries, 69
  as intermediate essential oil, 63
  for physical level, 34
  quick reference, 188
  subtle properties of, 50

K

Kaminski, Patricia, 20
Kanuka, 174
Krieger, Dolores, 11
Kunz, Dora, 11

L

Lantana, 174
Larch, 174
Lavabre, Marcel, 3
Lavender
  for affecting consciousness, 71
  as basic essential oil, 62
  in baths, 7
  to clear and cleans, 67
  for Combing & Smoothing
      technique, 155
  in cosmetic applications, 1
  for Filling technique, 153
  for Forehead Spread technique, 149
  to increase awareness
      of healing energy, 22
  in medical applications, 1
  for Open Toes/Close Toes
      technique, 148
  for positive energy, 68
  safety of, 8
  for stress relief, 118

quick reference, 188
subtle properties of, 50
undiluted, 6
Lemon
    as basic essential oil, 62
    to clear and cleanse, 67, 140
    for energy boundaries,
    quick reference, 188
    subtle properties of, 51
Lemongrass, 51
Leptospermum, 174
Lime, 51
Limits, respecting, 143
Listening, active, 144
"Listening to an Essential Oil"
    exercise, 35
    fill-in form, 185
Lovage, 174

M

Magnolia, 174
Mandarin, 52
Mangoginger, 174
Marjoram
    as intermediate essential oil, 63
    quick reference, 188
    to relieve stress, 118
    subtle properties of, 52
Massage, 7
    for stress relief, 118
Mastic, 174
Maury, Margarite, 3
Meadowsweet, 175
Melissa,
    as advanced essential oil, 63
    quick reference, 188
    subtle properties of, 53
Mental body, 19
Mental well-being, 110
Merton, Thomas, 127
Mimosa, 175
Misters
    body, 8
    common method, 5
Misting
    definition of, 66
    working with energy centers, 73

Monarda, 175
Montaque, Ashley, 20
Mugwort, 8
Music, 33, 109, 110, 111, 113, 130,
    131, 136
Myrrh
    as advanced essential oil, 64
    quick reference, 188
    subtle properties of, 53
Myrtle, 175

N

Narcissus, 175
National Association of Holistic
    Aromatherapy (NAHA), 3
Native Americans, 34
Neroli
    as intermediate essential oil, 63
    in cosmetic applications, 1
    for positive energy, 68
    quick reference, 188
    to relieve stress, 118
    subtle properties of, 54
    to support creativity, 130
Niaouli, 175
Nigella Seeds, 175
Nutmeg, 54

O

Oakmoss
    as advanced essential oil, 64
    quick reference, 188
    subtle properties of, 54
Open-ended questions, 144
Open Toes and Close Toes
    technique, 146-148
    aromatherapy, subtle, for, 147
    quick reference, 179
    visualization & color exercise for, 148
Opopanax, 175
Orange, color of, 28
Orange, essential oil of
    for affecting consciousness, 71
    as basic essential oil, 62
    for Filling technique, 153
    for positive energy, 68
    quick reference, 188

to relieve stress, 118
subtle properties of, 55
Oxides, 6

P

Palmarosa
    for Combing & Smoothing
        technique, 155
    as intermediate essential oil, 63
    for Open Toes/Close Toes
        technique, 148
    quick reference, 188
    subtle properties of, 55
Paraphrasing, 144
Pastinak, 175
Patchouli
    as intermediate essential oil, 63
    quick reference, 188
    subtle properties of, 56
    to support creativity, 130
Pendulum
    to assess energy centers, 125
    using a, 125
Pennyroyal, 8
Peppermint
    as basic essential oil, 62
    avoid with children, 10
    for indigestion, 152
    quick reference, 188
    subtle properties of, 56
Persuasive resonance, 33
Petitgrain
    for positive energy, 68
    subtle properties of, 56
Physical well-being, 108
Pine
    for affecting consciousness, 71
    to clear and cleanse, 68
    for Filling technique, 153
    subtle properties of, 57
Pituitary gland, 6
Plant gestures and signatures, 34
Play, 105, 107, 110, 111, 135
Polarity Therapy, 11
Positive energy, to bring in, 68
    quick reference, 191
Positive energy blends, 68

Positive mind blend, 71
Pregnant, 9
Preparing your hands, 22
Preparing yourself, 21, 71

Q

Questions, open-ended, 144

R

Referrals, 145
Relationships, 15, 19, 21, 105, 107, 112
Relaxation Response Breath, 117
Relaxation, session for, 156
Relaxing Breath, 117
Rest, 105, 107, 108, **109**, 116, 134
Room spray, 7
Rose
    as basic essential oil, 62
    in baths, 7
    for Combing & Smoothing
        technique, 155
    in cosmetic applications, 1
    expense of, 4
    for positive energy, 68
    quick reference, 188
    subtle properties of, 57
    to support creativity, 130
Rosemary
    for affecting consciousness, 71
    as basic essential oil, 62
    to clear and cleanse, 68
    for Filling technique, 153
    for Forehead Spread technique, 148
    for positive energy, 68
    quick reference, 188
    subtle properties of, 58
Rosewood
    for Forehead Spread technique, 149
    as intermediate essential oil, 63
    for positive energy, 68
    quick reference, 188
    subtle properties of, 58
    to support creativity, 130

S

Sacred space, setting, 67, 155
Safe, session to feel, 158

Safety, essential oils and, 8-10
Sage, 34. See also Clary Sage
Sandalwood
    for affecting consciousness, 71
    as basic essential oil, 62
    for Forehead Spread technique, 149
    quick reference, 189
    subtle properties of, 59
Santolina, 176
Savory, Winter, 176
Schnaubelt, Kurt, 3
Second energy center (Sacral)
    affirmations for, 133
    to assist, quick reference, 193
    blends, 78
    colors and, 15, 28
    essential oils for, 77
    explanation of, 15
    imbalances in, 78
    strengthening, 135
    questions to assess, 122
Security, session for, 158
Sensing the Subtle Bodies, 24
Self-care
    assessing your energy centers for, 121
    essence of, 105
    exercises, 113, 126-141
    questionnaire, 105
    subtle energy for, xiv
    visualization technique, 129
Self-esteem, session for, 160
Senses, nourishment through, 130
Seventh energy center (Crown)
    affirmations for, 134
    to assist, quick reference, 194
    assessing, 123
    blends for, 96
    color and, 17, 29
    essential oils for, 94
    explanation of, 17
    imbalances in, 95
    positive actions for, 135
    questions to assess, 123
    quick reference for assisting, 194
    strengthening, 135
Showers, 128, 129
Sight, sense of, 33, 130, 131

Silence, 131
Simple Hold technique, 138, **149**
    aromatherapy for, 150
    positions for specific situations, 140
    for stress relief, 119
    quick reference, 179
    visualization and color exercise, 150
Sixth energy center (Brow, Third Eye)
    affirmations for, 134
    to assist, quick reference, 193
    assessing, 123
    blends for, 92-94
    color and, 17, 29
    essential oils for, 90
    explanation of, 17
    imbalances in, 92
    positive actions for, 135
    questions to assess, 123
    quick reference for assisting, 193
    strengthening, 135
Skin
    care, 1, 3, 8
    irritation, 9
    as liminal boundary, 20
Sleep, 105, 107, 108, **109**, 116
Smell, sense of, 5
Spikenard, 176
Spiritual body, 19
Spiritual guidance, ask for, 69, 192
Spiritual guidance blends, 69
Spiritual rejuvenation, session for, 162
Spiritual well-being, 112
Spruce
    as advanced essential oil, 64
    subtle properties of, 59
    quick reference, 189
St. John's Wort, 176
Stone, Randolph, 11
Stress
    bath for, 7
    energy center reaction to, 14
    essential oils to relieve, 118
    healing touch and, 21
    management questionnaire, 117
    massage for relieving mental, 8
    as a part of life, 114
    play and, 111

reduction and management, 115-119
reduction questionnaire, 116
session for, 156
techniques for coping with, 116
Stroking
definition of, 66
working with energy centers, 72
Study, 110
Subtle anatomy, 2, **13**, 33, 127, 137
to balance with Open Toes &
Close Toes technique, 146
creative activities and, 129
Subtle aromatherapy
ability to promote well-being, 65
aromatherapy referred to as, 2
intended to assist, xii
as vibrational medicine, 33
Subtle bodies, 2, 13, **18-20**, 33, 34
sensing, 24
Subtle energy, 13
Subtle energy terminology, 30
Subtle energy medicine, 12
Subtle energy therapy
applications for using essential
oils in, 66
to balance energy centers & subtle
bodies, 127
basic hand positions for, 145-155
benefits of, 11
color and, 28
examples of, 11
to help common imbalances, 181-183
historic use of, xvi
intention and, 27
intuition and, 29
principles of, 11
traditional use of, 33
as vibrational medicine, 33
visualization and, 27
Subtle energy therapy sessions
for relieving aches, 157
after, 163
basic hand positions for, 145-155
for common physical imbalances, 181
for common psychological
imbalances, 182

for common spiritual imbalances, 183
for confidence and
self-esteem, 160
to enhance creativity, 159
for positive communication, 161
ending, 162
for energizing, 157
giving, 155
for a joyful heart, 160
for relaxation and stress relief, 156
preparing to give, 155
to feel safe and secure, 158
for spiritual rejuvenation, 162
Subtle properties
determined, 33
of essential oils, 37-62
indicators of, 34
of uncommon essential oils, 169

T

Tansy, 8
Tarragon, 177
Taste, sense of, 33, 130, **131**
Tea Tree
in medical applications, 1
safety of, 8
subtle properties of, 60
undiluted, 6
Tending Touch exercise, 136
Therapeutic Touch, 11
Third energy center (Solar Plexus)
affirmation for, 133
to assist, quick reference, 193
blends, 82
color and, 16, 29
essential oils for, 80
explanation of, 16
imbalances in, 81
strengthening, 135
questions to assess, 122
Thuja, 8
Thyme
as advanced essential oil, 64
quick reference, 189
subtle properties of, 60
Tisserand, Robert, 3

Tolu-balsam, 176
Touch. See also Hands
    anointing, 66
    compassionate, 20, 145
    as human need, 20
    massage, 7
    sense of, 33
Touch Research Institute, 20
Traditional Chinese Medicine (TCM), 20
Tuberose, 177

U
Uncommon essential oils, 169-177

V
Valerian, 177
Valnet, Jean, 2
Van Der Post, Lauren, 5
Vega, Selene, 13
Verbena, Lemon, 6, 177
Vetiver
    as intermediate essential oil, 63
    for Combing & Smoothing
        technique, 155
    for Open Toes/Close Toes, 148
    quick reference, 189
    subtle properties of, 60
Vibrational Medicine, 18, **33**, 163
Violet, essential oil, 177
Visualization, 27
Vital energy, 105, 130, 136

W
Well-being
    emotional, 111
    four dimensions of, 107
    mental, 110
    physical, 108
    promoted by essential oils, 1, 5
    promoted by subtle energy therapy, 11
    spiritual, 112
    touch and, 20
Wholistic, 11, **33**
Work, 110
Working with the energy centers, 72
Wormwood, 177

Y
Yarrow, Blue, 177
Ylang Ylang, 61

Made in the USA
Monee, IL
08 March 2022

92472357R00135